KU-319-981

An Encyclopaedia of Homoeopathy

**A comprehensive reference book and survey
of the subject from its beginnings to the
present day**

by
Trevor Smith
MA, MB, BChir, DPM, MFHom

THE BRITISH SCHOOL OF OSTEOPATHY
1-4 SUFFOLK ST., LONDON. SW1Y 4HG
TEL. 01-930 9254-8

Insight Editions
Worthing, Sussex

First Published 1983

© Trevor Smith 1983

This book is sold subject to the condition that it shall not, by
by way or trade or otherwise, be lent, hired out or otherwise
circulated without the publisher's prior consent in any form of
binding or cover other than in which it is published and
without a similar condition including this condition being
imposed on the subsequent purchaser

THE BRITISH SCHOOL OF OSTEOPATHY
1-4 SUFFOLK ST, LONDON SW1Y 4HG
TEL 01-930 9254-8

ISBN 946670 01 3

Printed and bound in Great Britain

Preface

Aims and Objectives
The reference book — clarifies and explains the following major areas of Homoeopathic interest.

1) The most important historical personalities and prescribers of the Homoeopathic scene of the last 150 years.

2) The common illnesses in outline with a brief list of the most relevent remedies.

3) The major remedies are listed and a brief outline is given of their remedies.

4) The essential areas of homoeopathic philosophy involving the approach and the process of describing are dealt with and contrasted with the conventional allopathic approach to the patient and his illness.

This book is dedicated with affectionate gratitude to the many patients who have worked patiently with me — accepting my limitations and fumblings with as much good spirit and grace as my more inspired moments. Their patience, humour and faith has been an example and source of inspiration and strength over the past 25 years.

Contents

Introduction

The book aims to give an overall account of homoeopathy in alphabetical reference form. It includes a review and up-dating of my thinking on key homoeopathic principles and the philosophy of the method. I have included biographical notes on the major historical and contemporary figures who have played a role in homoeopathic development and thinking since its inception. The choice of historical entries has been extended and enlarged as a result of lobbying colleagues for their list of the most significant and key personalities since Hahnemann, and I would like to express here my gratitude for their support and suggestions. Finally I have given the key-notes of the main remedies with a note on all the common major illness-conditions with a recommended list of remedies to consider when prescribing and in the choice of simillimum.

In this way I have tried to create an overall volume of greater general interest and reading on the subject which also has a practical usage. The notes on philosophy and historical background are intended for information and as guide-lines for discussion.

All cure is from within; medicines themselves do not cure — not even the homoeopathic ones. They only act by deeply mobilising within the individual pathways of vital reaction towards cure. What man has caused — in this context illness and disease — man can also cure. Often the key causative factor lies within the mind, undermining resistance and vitality. This vital reaction, really a movement of energy within the person, is in us all — if it can be mobilised. Without doubt, homoeopathy is one of the most important and effective tools to stimulate a curative response because it acts like a natural catalyst. Only in recent years has the inherent power of the remedies been more widely appreciated which is why the method has become more recognized by the patient.

But more doctors need to know and to appreciate homoeopathy. This is inevitably a slower process because medical education is still rooted in the synthetic and pharmaceutical approach of suppression of symptoms — ultimately of the individual, so that homoeopathy appears quite alien, unscientific and suspect.

Homoeopathy does not and cannot promise or guarantee that a cure will occur but it does promise a method of approach and a treatment of each person as an overall individual. It has genuine potential for cure provided that the method is not contraindicated or a conventional approach for a particular physical or mechanical problem more indicated and superior.

Homoeopathy offers what is best for the individual — even where it is not homoeopathy. This overall caring attitude is part, if not the essence of being holistic. An unbiased approach is essential where the patient and their needs come first and not the principles of any method or the need to prescribe whatever the problem.

Homoeopathy is a unique system of medicine with a wide range of potential and treatment and many of its therapeutic resources have not yet been fully recognized nor its benefits to the patient when prescribed in proper depth and potency. The method should not be abused by implying that it is indicated where other methods are better advised and of more value as this only does the method and the intelligence of the patient a disservice.

There is more to homoeopathy than just matching the symptom-picture of the patient to the toxic proving-profile of the remedy. The Law of Similars is quite fundamental and a guideline to prescribing but the experienced practitioner must also take the potency into account. The more recent high serial dilutions offer a greater dimension to homoeopathic thinking because in this form they are able to mobilise the most inflexible and defended parts of both mind and body.

Because of its action on temperament and attitudes as well as the physical it opens avenues of therapeutic possibility previously thought irreversible.

For the best results it is not sufficient to just guess at the correct potency or to prescribe by rule-of-thumb. A proper assessment must be made during the initial diagnostic consultation of the true level of primary disturbance. This should be discussed with the patient during the consultation-dialogue and then mobilised by the correct prescription at the right potency. It is the potency which determines the depth reached by the remedy. The latter specifies the areas of mobilisation. Having plumbed the depths during the consultation, or more often, allowing them to emerge spontaneously, the potency gives the correct weighting and depth to the remedy-line during treatment and this depth should be regularly re-appraised. The correct remedy may be the constitutional one or it may be a 'low', more pathological one, but whenever a high potency is chosen for whatever reason it should always be followed by a back-up consultation in about 2 weeks to provide essential support for the patient. At that time it may not be necessary to re-prescribe because improvement has occured. But where mobilisation is inadequate or gives rise to anxiety, there will be a need for extra reassurance and possibly a further remedy. This is the essence of good prescribing.

Homoeopathy should not be a last resort but prescribed early where indicated. It is hoped that this volume will provide a small contribution to the field of therapeutics and appreciation of the method and its potential.

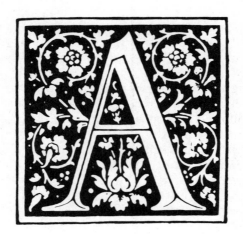

Abrasions and Cuts

Clean the wound with *Calendula* cream or tincture. If the patient is shocked give *Arnica* 30 hourly until there is improvement. Where the wound is dirty give *Hepar Sulph* or *Mercurius*. For a penetrating wound give *Ledum 6* or *Hypericum 6*. When there is a foreign body or the remnants of it in the wound, this must be removed immediately — either by the family or the nearest hospital casualty department.

Abscess

A painful inflammatory condition of the skin or other internal organ where there is swelling with heat, redness and pulsating pain causing restlessness and discomfort. In severe cases the abscess may become toxic, provoking drowsiness and fever, with a discharge of pus.

REMEDIES.

Anthracinum, Sulphur, Belladonna, Hepar Sulph, Silicea, Mercurius, according to the symptoms.

Accidents

When there is damage to tissues caused by trauma. Often these are the common first-aid conditions which occur in the home. *Arnica* is always the most important immediate remedy for shock. Any bleeding must be stopped by local pressure or tourniquet.

Where there has been a severe burn or scald give rescue remedy (Bach) — 5 drops every hour with *Arnica 30* in a single dose daily until recovery occurs. Give *Cantharis 6* or *Urtica Urens* for burns according to symptoms. If the condition is severe the patient must be urgently hospitalised in a specialised burns unit.

Accident-Proneness

The tendency to be frequently involved in one form of accident or another for underlying psychological reasons.
REMEDIES include:
Kali Carb when due to undue nervousness.
Lycopodium — when the person is always distracted or preoccupied and elsewhere — never listening or concentrating.
Baryta Carb when associated with the elderly.
Zincum Met where there is marked agitation.

Acidity

A sensation of bitterness or acidity in the stomach, causing discomfort often associated with flatulence, heartburn and indigestion.
REMEDIES
Mag Phos. 6, Lycopodium 6, Carbo Veg. 6 three times daily.

Acne

The common chronic skin affection of teenagers and young adults. The exact cause is unknown but major contributing factors are stress, hormonal imbalance, poor and unbalanced diet, particularly one too rich in starchy and refined sugars. If not corrected, the condition leads to permanent scarring in later years.
REMEDIES
Sulphur 6, Kali Brom 6, Graphites 6 (especially when the acne oozes a clear fluid). Where there is scarring use such remedies as *Thiosinaminum, Variolinum* or *Phytolacca.*

Aconitum Napellus (Monkshood)

One of the most acute remedies of all for colds and flu. It should be taken within the first 48 hours of onset. Especially indicated

4

when symptoms are those of fear, pain, apprehension, restlessness and fear of dying. The pains often follow exposure to wind, rain or cold. The typical subject for *Aconitum* is of florid complexion and solid, well-built frame.

Acrocyanosis

A condition of peripheral cyanosis with a red or bluish tint to the peripheral extremities. Associated with poor circulation and coldness.
REMEDIES
Lachesis 6, Carbo Veg 6, Agaricus 6.

Adhesions

These are a complication of either surgical intervention or previous infection. When healing occurs, scar fibrous tissue is laid down in the area affected causing distortion, sometimes blockage with interference to normal functioning.
REMEDIES
Thiosinaminum, Graphites, Phytolacca, Staphysagria, Bellis perennis.

Adolescent Depression

Depression of the teenage years, sometimes severe. There is often withdrawal from others into fantasy and a preoccupation with sexual problems, body imagery, hypochondriasis and guilt — often about masturbation.
REMEDIES
Natrum Mur, Murex, Lycopodium.

Aerophagy

The common habit in certain children and adults of constantly swallowing air when eating or on other occasions. This leads to symptoms of flatulence, fullness, indigestion and discomfort generally. Often the aerophagy is quite unconscious.
REMEDIES
Carbo Veg, Lycopodium 6 and *Arg. Nit. 6.*

5

Aesculus Hippocastanum (Horse Chestnut)

Mainly a remedy for problems of the rectum and anal areas. Pain, congestion and discomfort are marked from a combination of haemorrhoids and chronic constipation. Anal prolapse, anal itching, sharp sudden deep rectal pain and discomfort. Of value for chronic conditions in the area.

Aethusa (Fool's Parsley)

One of the major remedies for milk allergy in infants and children. Milk cannot be tolerated in any form provoking vomiting soon after swallowing. The vomit is usually violent and projectile with curds which are 'shot out' as from a canon. In adults it is useful when there is an allergic condition to dairy products.

Agaricus Amanita (Amanita Toad Stool)

Indicated in confusional states including chronic alcoholism. Of special value in circulatory problems and helpful in chilblains or frost bite where there are red areas of burning itching and swelling of fingers and toes. The extremities are cold, blue and painful.

Agarophobia

Fear and panic at going out of doors alone or into any busy unfamiliar area. Usually there is a restricted feeling and fear of being held-up or delayed. All the symptoms are better for company and security. Having to wait in a queue, at a check-out point or traffic-light can often worsen anxiety. The cause is always profoundly psychological.
REMEDIES
Natrum Mur, Lycopodium, Arg. Nit, Pulsatilla.

Aggravation-of Symptoms

This may occur in the course of homoeopathic treatment especially in the early stages. It often happens where the underlying problem has been pushed down or suppressed over a period of time so that it is not readily available to the remedy's action. Homoeopathy seems to worsen the condition as it brings it out to the surface. In this way it can be more easily and readily dealt with

6

by the body as vital energy flows into the region making it more accessible to cure. Such aggravations are usually only transient aspects of early homoeopathic treatment and understood by the patient as such because they do not undermine the more general and important improved sense of well-being.

Ageing Problems

These are many and varied but all centre around the general problem of degenerative changes. The commonest symptoms are loss of memory, confusion, anxiety and agitation, insomnia, arthritis, weakness.

REMEDIES
Baryta carb, Opium, Carbo Veg, Sulphur.

Agitation

The state of mental unrest, with fidgety restlessness usually due to internal turmoil and anxiety. Insomnia is also commonly present.

REMEDIES
Zinc Met. when the restlessness is mainly of the feet.
Arg. Nit. when underlying panic and fear is the major cause
Lycopodium, where fear of an anticipated event provokes unrest.

Agnus Castus (Chaste Tree)

Although particularly effectively in the sexual sphere, it is a remedy generally for loss of vigour and drive where there is depression, disinterest and a weak response generally. For the male it is invaluable for impotence, weakness and inadequacy (compare Silicea). In the female it has a similar role where there is a diminished libidinal interest and activity or sterility.

Air-Sickness

Symptoms of malaise, usually sickness, nausea, excessive salivation and dizzyness occur when travelling by plane.

REMEDIES.
Cocculus when dizzyness and nausea are marked,
Berberis when the nausea occurs in an air-pocket with sudden downard movement.
Pulsatilla when there is a psychological element strongly present

7

with apprehension made worse by noise or vibration.

Alcoholism

The common social addictive problem with excessive alcohol
intake to compensate for feelings of underlying psychological
inadequacy. There is often a strongly positive response to
homoeopathy and remedies as *Nux. Vom, Avena Sat* may be
required in high potency together with the constitutional
prescription.

Aletris Farinosa (Stargrass)

The remedy acts strongly upon the digestive system and
reproductive organs. Indigestion, colicy pains and flatulence with
nausea is common. The appetite is nil and the sight or thought of
food stimulates nausea. Vomiting of pregnancy. The menstrual
periods are heavy and excessive with clots and severe colicy pains.
Anaemia, exhaustion, recurrent miscarriages.

Allen, Henry C. M.D. (1836-1909)

The early American homoeopathic physician and writer. He first
(with Swan) described provings of Lueticum in The Materia
Medica of the nosodes with provings of the X-Ray (Boericke and
Tafel Phil. 1910).
Major writings include:
*Keynotes with Nosodes, Important Nosodes, Materia Medica of
the Nosodes, The therapeutics of Intermittent Fever.*

Allen, Timothy Field M.D. (1937–1902)

The emminent American homoeopath, best known for his
Encyclopædia of Pure Materia Medica in 10 volumes and still a
standard quoted reference book. He worked mainly in Brooklyn,
N.Y., where he was in practise. Born in Westminster, Vermont, he
was son of a doctor and also known as an organist and composer.
In 1867 he became professor of anatomy at the New York
homoeopathic college and in 1871 professor of therapeutics and
materia medica. He was also director of the New York
homoeopathic asylum for the insane. Allen worked as co-editor
of the New York Journal of Homoeopathy.

8

Major writings include:
1874 *Encyclopædia of Pure Materia Medica*
1876 *Opthalmic Therapeutics*
1878 *The effects of Lead on healthy individuals*
1880 *A general symptom register of Homoeopathic Materia Medica*
1889 *A handbook of Materia Medica and Homoeopathic Therapeutics.*

Allergy

There is an acute antibody-reaction by the body to a protein element in the irritant which is treated as a foreign body stimulating an inflammatory reaction. This may occur in asthma, hay-fever or following a bee or wasp sting. *Urtica Urens 6* given hourly in the acute attack is helpful to relieve swelling and irritation.

Allium Cepa (onion)

The major symptoms of this useful remedy are those of the common cold with a streaming nasal watery discharge, itchy watering eyes and acute nasal catarrh, irritation and exhaustion. Useful in hay-fever.

Allopathic

The system of conventional medicine which differs from homoeopathy by treating symptoms with their opposite in order to suppress them. When the patient is hot he is given something to cool him down. When in pain — something to eradicate the pain and when agitated, a drug to calm him down. When over-calmed he is then given another drug to stimulate. This is in direct contrast to the Homoeopathic approach which gives a 'like' remedy based on the Theory of Similars to stimulate natural vital energy in the area affected.

Aloe (the common aloe)

Mainly a rectal remedy for haemorrhoidal problems. There is restlessness and irritability. Chronic colicy diarrhoeal problems with a tendency to soiling. Haemorrhoidal conditions which protrude and prolapse with much pain, congestion and burning.

Alopoecia

Loss of hair in circular or irregular patches in either sex. Male-pattern baldness is hereditary in origin, but stress and hormonal imbalance is causative in other cases. More rarely the condition is complete and may occur in children or adults — the cause unknown.

REMEDIES
Lycopodium, Vinca Minor 6.

Alternative Medicine

Dr. Marjorie Blackie always said that Homoeopathie was 'the' alternative medicine. It certainly offers a viable alternative to the conventional prescription for both patients and physician alike. Much of conventional medicine is laboratory-based and largely synthetic, using products which suppress rather than conserve vital energy. Over-prescribing has become increasingly common and is responsible for a lot of the present dissatisfaction with the health service approach to community health.

Alumina (the metal Aluminium — as its oxide)

Main indications are chronic and absolute constipation — the type where manual removal of faeces may be required, eczema and 'itchy eyes'. The use of aluminium utensils in the kitchen should be systematically avoided by all homoeopathic users.

Ammonium Muriaticum (Sal Ammoniac)

A remedy for paralysing exhausting symptoms nearly always worse first thing in the mornings. The make-up is sluggish, oedematous and obese often with slowness in all areas of the digestive system. Depression, headache, especially at the root of the nose. The head feels bruised. Scalp irritation and chronic problems of scalp-eczema and dandruff.

Ammonium Phos. (Phosphate of Ammonia)

The titration of the organic salt, first proved by Voigt. It is a remedy for chronic problems, particularly recurrent gout, poor circulation and facial paralysis.

Acts on the hands and feet where there are chronic gouty and arthritic problems with swelling, nodular formation and pain.

10

Amnesia

Loss of memory associated with fatigue and poor concentration (*lycopodium*). Where there is a history of head injury, however remote, that set off the problem then *Helleborus* should be considered. When the cause has been shock of any kind give *Arnica*. Hysterical amnesia responds well to *Ignatia*. If due to senility then *Baryta Carb* may improve the condition.

Amyl Nitrosum (Amyl Nitrate)

A major remedy for flashes of heat and tension in the head with anxiety and sweating with palpitations. Such symptoms occur at the menopause and afterwards causing distress. They can also occur in a younger person — either male or female with general over-sensitivity and painful sweating and sensations of heat and head fullness. The remedy has tachycardia, pulse irregularity and chest pain of the anginal type radiating down the arm or up into the neck area. Flushing, throbbing and violent heart-beating is the key to prescribing. (Compare *Belladonna*).

Anacardium Orientale (Marking Nut)

A remedy for chronic digestive problems associated with pain and fullness after meals, but relieved by further eating. Constipation is severe and chronic. There are many odd and bizarre and hypochondriacal facets to the remedy in particular the not uncommon symptom of the inside or uterus being 'blocked by a plug', or of a girdle or a hoop encircling the body. Weakness is associated. The bizarre ideas are sometimes psychotic and delusional.

Anaemia

There is deficiency of the iron-containing blood element haemo-globin which binds and transports oxygen to the cells. When this is lacking, all the typical symptoms of exhaustion, pallor and shortness of breath are seen. The cause may be haemorrhage from a variety of causes, particularly heavy menstrual loss. It can occur in pregnancy and also from dietary insufficiency.

REMEDY

Ferrum Met. is indicated but the underlying cause must always be diagnosed and treated.

11

Angina Pectoris

There is heavy constricting pain across the chest and sometimes up into the neck or down the arms. The cause is always due to insufficient blood supply to the heart usually due to arterio-schlerosis of the coronary arteries supplying the heart muscle. Pain is typically worse for physical effort and relieved by rest.
REMEDIES
Latrodectus, Cactus, Nux Vomica, Arsenicam Alb.

Animal Experiments

These are not used in the testing or 'proving' of homoeopathic remedies — traditionally carried out on healthy, symptom-free volunteers. In recent years a few European animal research experiments have been carried out to demonstrate the efficiency of certain remedies in potency on the regeneration of liver-cells poisoned by a toxic substance. In general these are the exception and homoeopathy is based solely on symptoms recorded by the healthy human — which makes up the repertory.

Anorexia Nervosa

The common emotional illness of adolescent girls where there is a preoccupation with weight loss, body image and compulsive food intake. Dieting may be severe, to the extent that health and life is threatened. The underlying psychological attitudes in both patient and family must be explored.
REMEDIES
Pulsatilla, Natrum Mur, Sulphur.

Anthracinum (Anthrax)

Prepared from the anthrax-infected spleen of sheep, and first introduced by Swann. It is an important and valuable remedy, particularly where there are severe infections, boils or carbuncles with pus and burning pains.

Antidotes to Homoeopathic Remedies

On rare occasions a patient is unable to tolerate the homoeopathic vital reaction because it is too strong, or the remedy may severely bring to the surface an earlier problem, so that it is felt to be overwhelming. In such cases the remedy can be neutralised or antidoted by its specific antidote.

In most cases *Sulphur* can be used to neutralise a remedy given unwisely after an improvement and prematurely so that there is a reaction — perhaps a proving symptom in a sensitive person, instead of leaving the single dose to complete the cure.

Antimonium Taricum (Tartar Emetic)

An acute remedy for inflammatory conditions, particularly effective in chest conditions where there is an accumulation of fluid and a loud rattling cough with laboured breathing as in asthma or bronchitis.

Anxiety States

The increasingly common psychological state of fear and insecurity not usually linked to an external event yet sufficient to provoke a severe response.

REMEDIES

Argentum Nit. when associated with fear.

Ignatia when linked with grief.

Natrum Mur where there is marked tension.

Pulsatilla useful for marked tearfulness.

Nux vom or *Sepia* for associated snappy irritability.

Lycopodium for marked hypochondriacal tendencies.

Aphasia (post stroke)

Loss of speech following a stroke. *Arnica 30* three times daily is recommended until improvement occurs.

Apis (The Hive Bee)

Source is the whole crushed bee. The action is rapid and dramatic, particularly indicated for acute condition with swelling, restlessness, redness, stinging pain, itching, and acute discomfort. A characteristic of the remedy is the marked absence of any desire to pass water and the lack of thirst (*Pulsatilla*).

Apomorphinum (The morphine alkaloid derivative)

A remedy to be considered for all states of severe and chronic vomiting sometimes without nausea. Sweating, fainting and weakness with giddyness is characteristic. Of value in alcoholism, drug addiction and abuse, vomiting of pregnancy.

Appetite Excess

There is an excessive and constant craving to eat or to pick at food at any opportunity, the appetite never appeased. The underlying reason is often one of stress and the tension turns to food, particularly sweet foods for comfort and relief. In chronic miasmic disease of the Psora type it is a particular feature when *Sulphur* may be indicated. In other cases the craving is for sweet things like *chocolate* where *Lycopodium* is the best remedy. Salt is also often taken excessively indicating *Natrum Mur* as a possible remedy. Once the underlying causative factors are clear then *Phytolacca Berry* is useful to control the appetite craving.

Appetite Loss

The loss of desire or interest in food. This may be a symptom of many acute conditions — often of infection during the incubation stage of measles or chicken pox or where there is any fever. It is also common in many of the more chronic debilitating illnesses as glandular fever and influenza. After Flu' *Cadmium Phos 6* is particularly helpful and for more general conditions of appetite loss *Kali Phos. 6* is helpful.

Argentum Nitricum (Silver Nitrate)

Nitrate of silver in titrated solution. Its main indications are for panic and anxiety states, particularly of the agarophobic type. There is great fear of failure and of the criticism by others as with a public speaking engagement, examination, interview or stage fright. The remedy always has the most absolute intolerance of heat of any kind (*Pulsatilla*) and abdominal flatulence and distension is commonly present. (*Carbo veg, Lycopodium*).

Arnica (Leopard's Bane)

Arnica takes its source from the Fall-kraut grown in the Alps at altitudes over 5,000 feet. It is one of the most useful and fundamental of all homoeopathic remedies and should be present in every family medical chest. its action is specific for bruising and shock and it is the major remedy for sprains with pain, inflammation and swelling. Shock from any cause, as after childbirth or dental extraction. Both respond well reducing recovery time and side-effects. When there has been a trauma of any kind — forceps at childbirth, an accident or injury and both before and after surgery, then *Arnica* makes the passage more comfortable and the recovery period shorter.

Arsenicum Alb (White trioxide of Arsenic)

Source is White arsenic oxide in homoeopathic potency. One of the polycrest remedies of multiple action, it is an acute remedy acting particularly on the chest and alimentary tract where there is restlessness, burning pains, craving for heat, chillyness, breathlessness or diarrhoea. Like *Arnica* it is one of the most useful of the homoeopathic remedies and should be in every family medical box in the home and taken on holidays, for emergency use.

Arteriosclerosis

Hardening of the arteries of the elderly, increasingly present in younger age groups as discovered at autopsies of U.S. Marine combat troops of the Korean war. The incidence was surprisingly high — some 30% in young soldiers. It is usually associated with diets high in animal fat and cholestrol but the cause is still largely unknown and stress may also be an important underlying cause.
REMEDIES
Baryta Carb, Carbo Veg, Cactus, Agaricus, the individual Constitutional remedy.

Arthritis

This may be osteo-arthritic or rheumatoid type. The former is due basically to wear and tear and may involve any joint, but it is particularly the large joints of knee, hip or spine which are most affected.

15

REMEDIES.

Causticum is indicated for certain types of neck arthritis.
Sanguinaria for arthritis of the shoulder joint and
Rhus Tox where there is stiffness, better for movement and heat, worse for damp.
Bryonia is called for when symptoms are aggravated by heat and movement.
Rheumatoid arthritis is an allergic condition, inflammatory in type which affects a younger age group and often smaller joints initially.
Apis is indicated for painful swelling.
Belladonna for redness, heat and swelling with pain.
Causticum when there is paralysis and wasting.
Medorrhinum for more chronic intractable conditions.

Asafoetida (Stinkasand)

Mainly a remedy for chronic hysterical problems often with a depressive origin to them. Chronic indigestion with aerophagy, flatulence, distention. An impression of having a lump in the throat (*Nat. Mur*). Variability of all symptoms and of mental attitudes generally. (*Pulsatilla*).

Asthma

The common condition of acute bronchospasm which can occur at any age but most commonly in childhood. The condition may be acute or chronic with marked shortness of breath, wheezing, apprehension and restlessness. Asthma often has a familial tendency to involve the shy sensitive personality with allergic tendencies.
REMEDIES.
Medorrhinum, Arsenicum, Kali Carb, Tub Bov, Phosphorus.

Aurum metallicum (the metal Gold)

A remedy which is especially indicated for chronic or recurrent depressive problems with suicidal despair or impulses present. There are many cardiac problems associated with palpitations, angina pectoris and often severe painful arthritic conditions as severe hip and knee disability. It is a remedy of immense importance and value.

16

Avena Sativa (the Oat)

Made from a tincture of the fresh flowering whole plant. Indications are extreme nervous prostration, impotence, palpitations, lack of concentration, insomnia. It is a useful remedy in drug addiction and alcoholism.

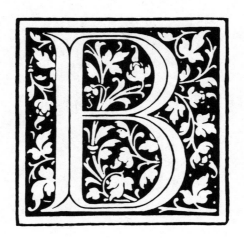

Baby — problems of

These respond well to the correct homoeopathic prescription. A clear diagnosis must be made in every case of the cause of each symptom.

REMEDIES:

Berberis 6. — Cries when put down.

Chamomilla 6 — Cries from anger when teething. Not thriving or failing to gain weight needs careful consideration and diagnosis.

Silicea 6 — Excessive wind.

Carbo Veg 6, mainly flatulence with abdominal distention (*Lycopodium*).

Aethusa 6 — Projectile vomiting.

Backward Child

The child is retarded in development and attaining normal expected milestones — both physically and mentally for his age. The causes are many, often obscure. These include constitutional or familial factors, mainly miasmic in type, especially psora, (see section) trauma, birth trauma, or infection during the early months of pregnancy. There may be a physical congenital deformity of the heart or vascular system. Down's Syndrome (mongolism) is another common factor.

REMEDIES

Nat. Mur for the difficult backward with behaviour problems, late in walking and with a tendency to sleep-walking.

Baryta Carb, more indicated for the dull, heavily built child, obviously slow and backward, looking more 'mental' and a tendency to enlarged glands and sore throats.
Medorrhinum for Down's syndrome (mongolism).
Tub. Bov. for children spiteful and resentful but always better for travelling.
Staphisagria where the child is extremely resentful but vulnerable and easily hurt and sensitive.
Capsicum for the backward child who is always homesick.

Backache

Lumbago is low back ache due to a combination of cold or damp together with muscle spasm. It is very painful and incapacitating. Sacro-iliac strain is ligamental strain from strain and effort with local tenderness, aching pain and sometimes sciatic pain. A prolapsed intervertebral disc often causes very severe, sometimes paralysing pain — usually incapacitating. Vertebral displacement from whatever cause is a mechanical problem that needs osteopathic correction initially. It often causes shortening of one leg and 'tilting' of the pelvis. One shoe may need adjusting.
REMEDIES
Rhus Tox, Bryonia, Medorrhinum, Sulphur, Causticum, Ruta, Nux. Vom, Natrum Mur, Radium Brom.

Balance (Internal)

This is an essential aspect of health especially at a psychological level. It is often only after internal harmony has been upset by stress, shock or poor nutrition — diminishing resistance and the vital force that illness occurs. The tissues quickly become vulnerable to invasion and illness as their intrinsic vitality is lessened. Symptoms often only appear at a much later stage, although malaise, fatigue, exhaustion and irritability are common early manifestations.

Barriers to Cure

These are relevant when the homoeopathic remedy fails to effect the expected vital response. There may be antidoting of the remedies by the use of an allopathic suppressant treatment at the same time as the homoeopathic one — from a steroid or antibiotic. The excessive use of coffee, tea or cigarettes can reduce the efficiency of the remedy. The remedy may have been neutralised and made ineffective by storage in excessive sunlight or heat, near camphor or strong perfumes. Excessive handling of the remedies undermines their efficiency. An underlying miasm may be present especially in chronic disease and make the expected treatement less efficient. Sometimes the patient themselves, if constantly taking homoeopathic remedies based on unwise self-prescribing, as soon as there is a symptom, prevents the prescribed remedy from being efficient. A final factor and an important one is that there is a mechanical barrier to cure, which requires either manipulation or surgery to relieve it.

Bed Wetting (enuresis)

There is a lack of normal control over bladder-functioning by the growing child at the time expected so that bed-wetting continues uncontrollably, often into the teens. It is far commoner in boys than girls. The condition may have existed since infancy, bladder-control never attained or in some conditions it was established early and then lost following a psychological shock or threat to security — as with a new baby.
REMEDIES
Lycopodium, Equisetum, Pulsatilla, Calc. Carb.

Belladonna (Deadly Nightshade)

The acute remedy for inflammatory conditions marked by heat, redness, pain, tenderness senstivity and restlessness. The condition may affect the ears with acute otitis media, the throat with acute tonsillitis or the skin with scarlet fever. The sensitivity is such that the very least jarring movement or draught of cold air provokes extreme irritation and an aggravation of the condition.

Bellis Perennis (Daisy)

A remedy for severe chronic sprains with damage to muscular fibres and tendons. Useful after *Arnica* when the condition persists and there is pain or discomfort and stiffness. For strain and tendon injury due to excessive effort, when caught off-balance or pain from a false movement or sudden cold or chill.

Fatigue, chill and swelling are marked and diagnostic.

Benjamin Alva M.D. (1884–1975)

The distinguished homoeopathic practitioner, formerly secretary-general of the International League and later president. Treasurer of the faculty council of the Royal London Homoeopathic Hospital for many years. A graduate of Sydney university, he was physician at the Royal London Hospital from 1923–56 with a special interest in dermatology. In 1958 he founded the Hahnemann Society.

Berberis Vulgaris (Barberry)

A major renal remedy. Pain and frequency are the major indications Renal colic is commonly relieved. There is often distortion of perspective so that typically other people look larger, or the head itself feels bigger enclosed in a tight-fitting cap. Often helpful in kidney stones.

Berridge, E. W., M.D. (   )

The American homoeopathic physician and graduate of Pennsylvania Homoeopathic college. Formerly resident medical officer to the Liverpool homoeopathic dispensary.
Major writings include:
1869 *Complete repertory of the Homoeopathic Materia Medica Diseases of the Eye.*
He is important because he was one of the earliest English homoeopaths, treating Skinner with high-potency remedies and instrumental in convincing him of the therapeutic merits of homoeopathy. Later he became Skinner's tutor.

Bites

If extensive and lacerating clean locally with *Calendula*, give *Arnica 30* followed by *staphisagria 6* hourly. Hospitalise the patient. When small and penetrating, give *Hypericum* and *Ledum*. Snake bites may require hospitalisation. When the bite is from a dog that is suspect of rabies give homoeopathic *Lyssin 30* daily until symptoms have subsided.

24

Blackie, Marjorie Grace, M.D. (1898–1981)

Probably the most well-known and respected homoeopath of recent years who has done so much to make Homoeopathy more widely appreciated in the past decades. Graduate of the Royal Free Hospital, Dean of the Faculty of Homoeopathy; great-neice of Compton-Burnett; physician to the Royal household since 1969 — her 50 years of practise were at all times a stimulating contact for both patients and students alike. She was a close colleague of Frank Bodman and they had remained close friends since the 20's when both served under Borland as house-physicians. She was an able lecturer, supporter of research, country lover, relaxing with a jig-saw-puzzle. A 'high' prescriber in Kentian traditions, she also taught the single, unrepeated-remedy traditional and pure approach to homoeopathy to the benefit of her many patients. Her Kensington fork-supper parties during the faculty meetings, must still be fresh in the memory of many. Her general approach to homoeopathy and style, was a joy to observe. She inaugurated the Blackie Research Trust and this continues her traditions. Many of her lectures are recorded on tape.

Her major writing is:
The Patient, not the Cure.

Bladder Problems

Infections — Pain, irritation — see Cystitis. Blockage — see Retention of urine, haemorrhage — see Haematuria. Stones — see Calculus section.

Bleeding (Haemorrhage)

Loss of blood from any part of the body — either of spontaneous or traumatic causation — other than normal menstrual loss. In all cases the flow must be stopped and any shock to the general condition must have priority. With bleeding from a wound or cut, arrest the flow by pressure locally. Give *Arnica* the shock and use *Calendula* locally.

REMEDIES.

For Nose bleeding or epistaxis:
Arnica 6 every few minutes until bleeding stops. When due to heat or raised blood pressure in a thick-set individual
Aconite 6. Where there is a recurrent tendency to nose-bleeds, and

25

the temperament passive, worse for heat, occuring in the latter part of the day, *Pulsatilla 6*. Bleeding from haemorrhoids indicates *Hammamelis 6*. *(Aesculus)*.

Blisters

Commonly due to friction from ill-fitting shoe or excessive local pressure or rubbing, causing damage to the skin.

Urtica is useful when there is much swelling with irritation.

Apis when there is less fluid with considerable sorness of surrounding tissues.

Cantharis where there is a persistance of burning discomfort, redness and pain.

When allergic in origin *Urtica 6*.

When following a bee or wasp sting *Apis*.

If part of the chicken pox rash use the nosode. *Mercurius 6* when infected.

mercurius 6.

Bodman, Francis Hervey (1900–1980) M.D.

The homoeopathic physician who studied with Blackie under Borland and Wheeler, working initially as a houseman to the Royal London Homoeopathic Hospital and later in Bristol where he established his practise. He had a D.P.M. psychiatric qualification as well as the homoeopathic degree and his stimulating and frequently erudite writings and communications always contained a sensitive awareness of the importance of the mentals and the psychological for the patient.

Boenninghausen, Clemens M.F. Von, M.D. (1785–1864)

Born in Heringhaven, Holland, he first qualified as a lawyer following family traditions and was only introduced to homoeopathy by chance. A serious fall led to a purulent tuberculous local condition of such a degree that in 1828, his life and health was despaired of. He was however cured by a friend and later colleague — Dr. Weihe, who used homoeopathy and converted him to the importance and significance of the method. From that time he became a most active supporter and promotor of homoeopathy through lectures and writings. His fame became such that in 1843 he was given a license by royal decree to practise homoeopathy, although not as a physician. In 1854 he received an honourary M.D. from the Cleveland Homoeopathic College. He corresonded regularly with Hahnemann throughout his life and they were close friends. Dr. Carol Dunham, the emminent homoeopath of that time was also a close friend and supporter. His major writings include:

1845 *Essay on the homoeopathic treatment of Intermittent Fever*
1847 *Boenninghausen's therapeutic pocket-book for homoeopathics.*
1847 *The sides of the body and drug affinities.*
1870 *The homoeopathic treatment of whooping cough.*
1873 *Homoeopathic therapia of intermittent and other fevers.*
Characteristics of homoeopathic remedies.

Boericke, Francis E., M.D. (1826–   )

Born in Glauchus Germany, Boericke settled in America where he became a lecturer at the Hahnemann medical staff college of Philadelphia. He is particularly known for establishing in Philadelphia the first and largest homoeopathic pharmacy in the U.S. In addition he formed the well known and highly regarded Boericke publishing company.

Boericke, William, M.D. (1849–1929)

The emminent American homoeopathic physician. Born in Czechoslovakia. He settled in Ohio at an early age. Graduate of the Philadelphia Medical College in 1876, he studied for a year in Vienna before moving to San Francisco where he worked as a homoeopath for 50 years. He was editor of the California Homoeopath, Founder of the Pacific Coast Journal of Homoeopathy in 1880 and editor until 1915. Co-founder of the Pacific Homoeopath Medical College in 1881 and professor of materia medica for 30 years. President of the California State Homoepathic Society.

His writings include:
Stepping Stones to Homoeopathic Health
The Materia Medica with Repertory
The Twelve Tissue Remedies (1890)
Principles of Homoeopathy

Management and Care of Children
His homoeopathic materia medica and repertory reached nine
editions and is still an everyday standard reference for many. He
also translated the important sixth edition of the Organon from
the complicated German text.

Boger C. M., M.D. (1861–1935)

The early homoeopathic practitioner.
His major writings include:
Synoptic Key to Materia Medica
Additions to Kent' Repertory
Boenninghausen's Characteristics
A Systematic Alphabetic repertory of homoeopathic remedies
Times of the remedies and the moon phases.

Bone Pains

This may be an aspect of injury or arthritis. The recommended
remedy is *Symphytum 6* three times daily.

Borax (Borate of Sodium)

The remedy has its major action on the intestinal tract with
nausea, vomiting, abdominal pains, and diarrhoea. Dizzyness
and sweating is marked. All symptoms are typically and
characteristically aggravated by downward motion in any form.

Borland, Douglas, M.D. (1885–1960)

The emminent teacher and prescriber who influenced so many
contemporary homoeopathic practitioners. Born in Glasgow and
a graduate from there, he was an outstanding teacher, prescriber
and lecturer. He was on the staff of the Royal London
Homoeopathic Hospital from 1913, later studying with Weir in
America under Kent on a Tyler scholarship. From 1945 he
became governor of the London Homoeopathic Hospital. He was
also president of the homoeopathic society. His monogram on
children's types is still widely read and referred to and has become
a classic. He was an advocate of high potency prescribing in
England and the important Kentian tradition of the single dose.

28

Bovista (Warted Puff-Ball)

The remedy for disordered speech including stammering and stuttering. There are many chronic skin problems with oozing eczemas, urticaria, corns and warts. The chronic eruptions have a crust and itch severely. All symptoms are worse for heat. (*Pulsatilla, Arg. Nit., Sulphur*).

Bowel Nosodes

Developed by Dr. John and Elizabeth Paterson who researched a series of nosodes from the non-lactose fermenting bowel organisms. They are enormously important in treatment, especially of chronic disease. The major bowel nosodes are *Morgan, Proteus, Gaertner, Dys. Co., Sycotic Co.*

Boyd, William Ernest, M.D. (1891–1955)

Dr. Boyd studied medicine, lived and practised in Glasgow throughout his life. He was a most eminent practitioner and thinker who combined the sensitivity of a physician with the practical approach of a research engineer. As a young man he was particularly impressed by the work of Gibson-Miller and eventually became committed to the homoeopathic method. He was physician to the Glasgow Homoeopathic hospital from 1920. Using concepts of electro-physics, he invented the emanometer to demonstrate the measurable force in homoeopathic potencies and to match this with 'emanations' from patient's tissues-fluids to select remedies.

He also carried out physiological and biochemical research and published many papers in the B.H.J., the major one being: *Biochemical and Biological Evidence of the Activity of High Potencies* (B.H.J. 1954).

Breasts — painful

When the problem is more in the nipples with acute inflammation take *Aconite 6* hourly until relief occurs. *Hepar Sulph* if the nipples are sore and cracked. Use *Merc Sol 6* where there is burning pain and marked swelling and deep-seated infection of the nipples. When pain is due to an abcess in the breast tissue, usually during lactation use the remedies as follows:

29

Bryonia when the breast is hard and painful.

Aconite for very acute cases.

Hepar Sulph 6 when there is obvious pus formation with throbbing pains and a raised temperature.

Sulphur 6 when the problem is at a more skin level generally with rubbing, chaffing and chapped skin.

Sulphur 6

Breathing difficulties

Usually these take the form of either shortness of breath or wheezing. In all cases the underlying reason must be very carefully diagnosed and any mechanical or obstructive cause dealt with. Chronic bronchitis and emphysema is one of the commonest causes and responds to remedies which stimulate the vital energies of the lungs. These include *Natrum Sulph, Bryonia, Phosphorus, Arsenicum, Ant. Tart.* Wheezing may be due to several factors including asthma, bronchitis or a foreign body. The causes must be carefully explored and an allergic factor dealt with by a specific remedy where appropriate.

REMEDIES

Phosphorus, Medorrhinum, House Dust, Kali Carb. Anxiety must also be taken into account as a possible trigger to the attacks.

Brittle nails

The nails are hard, without strength and are fragile tending to split and crack very easily — either downwards or across.

REMEDIES

Natrum Mur 6 — for hard, but brittle nails which break or crack easily.

Silicea 6 — especially where there is a tendency towards hang-nail infection of the finger tips.

Bronchitis

There is an infection, either acute or recurrent and chronic of the lining mucosal layer of the bronchial tubes. When chronic there may be mucosal thickening with yellow or white phlegm coughed-up. Asthma with bronchospasm is commonly associated.

REMEDIES

Bryonia, Hepar Sulph, Sulphur, Medorrhinum, Tub. Bov.

Bronchopneumonia

This is an acute inflammation of lung tissue, usually of the lung bases and often viral in origin, although sometimes bacterial in type. The onset can be very acute, often in an apparently fit strong person. There is a high temperature, shortness of breath and collapse.

When the condition involves the elderly the temperature may be normal, because of reduced vital reaction and antibiotics may be needed.

REMEDIES
Arsenicum, Lycopodium, Mercurius, Pyrogen, Ant. Tart.

Bryonia (Wild Hops)

The important remedy which has major action on the alimentary tract and mucous membrane generally — especially where there are acute conditions, with dryness and discomfort on movement. It also acts deeply on the joints. Pains are typically stich-like, and aggravated by both heat and movement and better for rest. The patient immobilises the affected area by lying on it, and the least movement is a cause of pain and irritation.

Bunions

There is chronic low-grade inflammation of the first or proximal metarso-phalangeal joint of the great toe associated with swelling, pain redness and painful thickening of the area. In most cases it is caused by tight, ill-designed and poor fitting shoes or poor posture. For an isolated bunion condition give

REMEDIES.
Silicea 6 three times daily.
Hekla Lava 6 is also useful to lessen the swelling once the acute inflammatory process has quietened down.
Rhus Tox 6 when the condition is part of a general arthritic or rheumatic process.

Burnett, James Compton, M.D. (1840–1901)

One of the most famous and prolific writers of all the English homoepaths of the last century. Great-uncle of Marjorie Blackie, his ability to communicate and explain the working principles and clinical results of homoeopathy did much to stimulate serious interest in the profession. He was an 'organ' prescriber and supporter of Rademacher's teachings.

His major writings include:

(1881) *The prevention of Congenital Malformation defects and disease.*

A series of essays and monographs, all classics, including 1882 *Natrum Muraticum, Gold, Cataract – causes and curability, Diseases of veins.*

1881 *The prevention of Congenital Malformation defects and disease.*

Burns

When severe give *Arnica 30* every hour for shock and hospitalise the patient immediately in a specialised burns unit. When only mild and localised, without shock, cover the area with vaseline gauze, give *Arnica 6* three times daily, or *Cantharis 6* for severe pain. *Hypericum* or *Calendula* cream can be applied locally. In more severe cases the area is best kept dry and exposed to clean air, the patient in bed and quiet. For blistering give *Urtica Urens 6* for redness and swelling *Belladonna 6* followed by *Sulphur 6* if the patient is not quickly made more comfortable in 24 hours. When extensive or in any doubt at all hospitalise immediately.

Cactus Grandiflorus (Night-blooming Cereus)

The important remedy for constricting pains — particularly of the heart in anginal conditions. The typical pain is like a tight-band and often there are palpitations and anxiety with a sense of oppression. Haemorrhages — both nose and anal.

Calendula Officinalis (Marigold)

The remedy for wounds, cuts, infection, boils or carbuncle. It may be given either locally or taken in potency — usually in the 6th potency. It acts to stimulate and provoke healing and lessens pus formation and infection. Stimulates drainage of any infected area and is basic to all first-aid treatment.

Calcarea Carbonica (Calcium Carbonate)

One of the most important of all the polycrest remedies. Indicated for chronic disease of the psora type with chill, sweating, lack of vital response and weakness.

Calcarea Hypophosphorosa (Hypophospite of Lime)

Of special value in the *calcarea* type of make-up with typical chill, pallor and coldness but with chronic arthritic conditions or rheumatism of the hands, which are damp, weak and cold always worse for humid chilly conditions.

Calcarea Iodata (Iodide of Lime)

For chronic glandular infections of the cervical region — especially tonsillar problems or goitre. Adenoidal chronic problems Fibrous tumours of the breast or uterus.

Calcarea Phosphorica (Phosphate of Lime)

For chronic conditions of weakness and pallor in a slim build and delicate make-up with marked weakness especially in the mental areas and where bone development has been interfered with by trauma or surgery. Buring pains of the *phosphorus* type with weakness and sweating give the diagnostic clue.

Calcarea Sulphurica (Plaster of Paris, Gypsum)

For chronic infected skin conditions in the *Calcarea* type of make-up which has the typical weakness, obesity and thick catarrhal discharges. Infection and pusy discharges, the skin dirty often greyish, but usually damp and chilly.

Camphora (Camphor)

An acute remedy for states of collapse with shock, pallor, chill and marked sweating, yet intolerance of any form of covering as a coat or blanket. Anxiety is marked with spasm and sometimes convulsions. Nausea, great coldness, low blood pressure, though less sweat than *Veratrum Alb*, which resembles it. May follow *Arnica* when it has failed to elicit a response.

Cannabis Indica (Hashish)

A remedy for mainly disturbed states of mind with dreamy unreality, hallucinations and disturbances of sensation and perspective. Useful in some psychotic conditions and for the ill-effects of drug-addiction — never well since that time, particularly after excessive maruanha. (Only obtainable on written prescription).

Cannabis Sativa (Hemp)

Mainly a remedy for ocular problems with lens opacity as cataract. There are also powerful irritating urinary symptoms with burning pains, urgency and spasm as severe cystitis or urethritis (Syotic Co) (only obtainable by written prescription).

Cantharis (Spanish Fly)

The remedy for acute irritating conditions of the mucous membrane, especially of the bladder where burning raw pains of excruciating intensity give the indication to prescribe. There is the most severe cystitis which gives no rest. It is active in any conditions of acute burning pain and this includes the skin as after a scald or burn or severe infective condition (compare *Belladonna.*)

Carbo Animalis (Animal Charcoal)

A remedy for the elderly, resembling Baryta Carb in many ways because of its ability to stimulate a vital reaction in broken-down chronic conditions with poor circulation and exhaustion. Chronic bronchitis and infection generally is common.

Carbo Vegetabilis (Vegetable Charcoal)

An important remedy for chornic digestive problems with flatulence, pain, gaseous formation and considerable discomfort. Weakness and collapse or when the reserves have been run-down by prolonged illness with weight loss. Slowness, uncertainty and fear marks much of the typical psychological reactions.

Carboneum Sulphuratum (Carbon Bisulphide)

A remedy for tremor, weakness and paralysis. Impotence. Particularly the eyes are affected with a variety of degenerative conditions including neuritis, central scotoma (black visual area), retinitis. Chronic digestive problems with flatulence and pain. Chronic constipation.

Carduus Marianus (St. Mary's Thistle)

One of the 'organ remedies' of Rademacher for problems of spleen and Liver disease, particularly jaundice or recurrent haemorrhages. The approach is more 'pathological' rather than based on the totality of the individual and is therefore not truly homoeopathic.

Care of the Remedies

The homoeopathic remedies should always be stored in a cool, dark medicine cupboard, preferably in a clean glass container not previously been used to store either allopathic or homoeopathic remedies. The remedies must be kept away from strong-smelling perfurmes or camphor which could neutralise the vitality of the potency and lead to ineffective results. When taking them, they should not be handled but taken from the lid as the remedy is impregnated on the outside layer of the tablet or pill.

Caries (dental)

The common tooth decay of adults or children with degeneration of the dental pulp due to chronic infection. Excessive quantities of sweet foods, convenience eating and poor dieting as well as hereditary weakness contribute to the condition, with diet being the major causative factor. The excess intake of certain vitamins can also mobilise calcium from the teeth, causing a deficiency and thereby undermining dental health.

REMEDIES
To prevent Caries and improve the dental resistance include *Calcarea Carb., Calc. Fluor, Silicea,* and the individual constitutional remedy.

Cataract

There is a gradual diminution of vision with increasing mistyness of sight. General health is not affected. It is a condition of the elderly due to either aging or trauma. The optical lens gradually becomes thickened and increasingly opaque. A comprehensive study on the subject was written by Compton-Burnett.

REMEDIES
Natrum Mur. 6, Cannabis Sat. 6, Silicea, Sulphur 6. All are important and play a role in treatment.

Catarrh

There is inflammatory thickening of the area affected involving the mucosal lining, causing an increased secretion of mucous which may be either clear, thick, or yellow-green in colour, according to the degree of infection and inflammation. Commonest areas are nasal and sinusitis catarrh, but the inflammation may also involve other areas as vagina, rectum, bladder, or middle ear.

REMEDIES

Pulsatilla 6 — For nasal catarrh and sinusitis.
The discharge variable in colour and consistency and aggravated by heat,
Bryonia, usually white or clear, with a lot of dryness and irritation in the area.
Kali Carb. 6 for the flabby build, far worsened by dry atmospheres and central heating.

Causation of Illness

These are many and complex, but in nearly all cases there has been a preceding stress factor to undermine vital resistance energy. Hahnemann placed a great deal of weight on such underlying psychological elements which he called the 'mentals' and from the start always emphasised that the key to cure lies within the mind. Where there is a severe illness it is common for the physician to find that the very deepest psychological elements of the personality have been shocked, disappointed or traumatised in some way — often several months before the onset of the illness. The resilience of the patient is undermined to such an extent that disease can penetrate, develop and take root. It is essential for cure that such mental factors emerge during treatment as they are effectively treated by homoeopathy and until they have come to the surface, the cure is often incomplete.

Cellulitis

The accumulation of fluid in the soft tissues and lymphatics immediately beneath the skin. The area is often unsightly and pitted. When stretched there is a typical 'peau d'orange' effect. Usually it is most noticeable in the upper thigh and buttock regions. Treatments recommended include diet, exercises.

REMEDIES

Natrum Mur 6, Apis 6, Urtica 6.

Centisimal scale of dilution

The principle of diluting one drop of the mother-substance in 99 drops of the dilutant fluid in serial dilution to obtain the homoeopathic potency. The sixth dilution commonly used in the U.K. is this serial dilution repeated six times, to give a dilution of 10^{-12} or one part in a billion.

Cerium Oxalicum (Oxalate of Cerium)

Introduced by Sir James Simpson. It is a specific remedy for congestion of the stomach mucosa causing nausea and vomiting. Especially useful for nausea of pregnancy and sea-sickness.

Chamomilla (Chamomile)

A remedy for pain, restlessness and irritability. Indicated for the young child that is teething, often with catarrh who refuses to be put down. Insomnia, impatience, crying, hot forehead, sweating and anger are typical.

Chelidonium Majus (Celandine)

A remedy which has an especial predisposition for liver and gall bladder. Jaundice and pain are characteristic. Pain is commonly of a bruised type — especially just under the right shoulder blade or in the gall-bladder area with tenderness. Drowsiness and nausea are frequent.

Chenopodium Anthelminticum (Jerusalem Oak)

For right-sided stroke with loss of consciousness and heavy snoring-like breathing. Pains beneath the right shoulder blade. Speech is typically lost.

Chloralum (Chloral Hydrate)

Indicated for urticaria, conjuctivitis, asthma, insomnia with an overactive mind. Delirium, confusional states. Congestion is a feature.

Cholecystitis

There is infection of the gall-bladder with associated pain and tenderness in the upper right abdomen. The condition may or may not be associated with gall stones. Symptoms include colicy pain — often severe, a raised temperature, sometimes jaundice with dark urine and pale stools when there is an obstruction.

REMEDIES

Chelidonium, Mag. Phos., Hepar Sulph, Sulph.

Cholera

The very severe bacterial infective condition of the bowel causing severe diarrhoea and collapse. It is often epidemic and in the past has caused much loss of life. There was a severe London outbreak in 1854 when treatment was far more successful using homoeopathic treatments than by conventional methods. Symptoms are severe watery diarrhoea, collapse and shock with vomiting and cramp.

REMEDIES

Arsenicum Alb. 6 for diarrhoea and collapse.

Camphor 6 for diarrhoea.

Veratrum Alb for severe cases of shock and collapse.

Cuprum Met 6 for cramps. Isolation and hospitalisation is essential whenever possible. Cases still occur with the speed of modern travel and because the disease is endemic in some tropical countries. Antibiotics are indicated where the disease is at all severe.

Chorea (St. Vitus Dance)

This disease of unknown origin is much less common than two or three generations ago when it was particularly frequent in hysterical female adolescents. At times the illness reached epidemic-like proportions with bizarre behaviour and multiple tic-like movements in whole communities. It is now rare — perhaps replaced by other problems as anorexia nervosa which in many ways is more dangerous.

REMEDIES

Stramonium — when there is great excitement.

Hyoxcyamus when there is destructive behaviour.

Natrum Mur, for an obvious emotional underlying problem.

41

Pulsatilla where the basic temperament is acquiescent and tearful. *Ignatia,* and *Zincum Met,* should also be considered.

Chronic disease.

Problems that are long-standing and recurrent over months or years in one form or another, forming well-recongnizable patterns of exhaustion, with a variety of physical psychological symptoms. The obviously indicated remedy gives but temporary relief and is ultimately ineffective whatever potency is used, and it is in these conditions that Hahnemann advocated the use of the nosode to effect a change in static vital energy response. He developed his classical treatise on chronic disease (1828) and theory of miasms with especially psora being a prime factor in causing energy-stagnation in depth. There has been a lot of disagreement and dispute as to the reality and value of the psora concept. But undoubtedly it is of enormous help still in appraising chronic problems and how best to treat them whether one accepts or not the causation of psora as originating with suppression of the 'itch' or scabies. The Bach and Paterson bowel nosodes have proved to be of value in such conditions and are worthy of study in order to extend the range of the therapeutic spectrum.

Cimicifuga Racemosa (Black Snake Root)

Great depression with agitation, maniac restlessness and talking. There are many uterine problems with pain, irregular periods. Recurrent miscarriage at the 3rd month. Puerperal Psychosis.

Cina (Worm Seed)

The important childrens remedy particularly of value in threadworm infection with irritation, fits, grinding of teeth, nightmares, nose picking and anal irritation at night. A dry chronic tickling cough in the mornings is characteristic.

Cinnamonum (Cinnamon)

A remedy for haemorrhage — as with nose bleeds. Always worse for exertion. It also has a role in certain hysterical problems with conversion symptoms in the gastric area and chronic vomiting. Weakness with bone pains are typical.

Circulatory problems

In most cases the blood supply to the periphery — fingers, hands and feet — is poor so that they are cold on the warmest day, the fingers sometimes white or blue. Cramps may be painful. The problem can occur at any age, the cause often hereditary or familial. In the elderly the cause may be due to arterioschlerosis. Intermittent claudication is cramp in the calf muscles on effort and occurs in the young adult associated with excessive cigarette smoking or in an older age group from hardening of the arteries. The pain goes with rest resembling angina and is due to insufficient blood supply to the local muscles.

REMEDIES

Silicea 6, Lycopodium 6, Carbo veg 6, Hammamelis 6, Baryta Carb 6, Agaricus 6.

Cirrhosis of the Liver

Usually a chronic condition with inflammatory disease of the liver cells leading to degeneration and eventual fibrosis. The causes are many but there has often been toxic irritation of the liver stimulating the breakdown of normal cell function and health. Commonest causes are chronic alcoholism due to the toxic action of alcohol on the liver cells and aggravated by the lack of essential vitamins in the diet. Toxic poisons, especially carbon tetrachloride used in dry cleaning, or following viral infection, particularly hepatitis has become an increasingly common cause. A cirrhosis-like condition with acute liver atrophy or fibrosis of essential functioning hepatic cells can occur as a complication and side-effect of certain synthetic drug treatments. The underlying cause must be treated when possible during the acute phase. Hospitalisation may be required.

REMEDIES

Phosphorus, Nux. vom.

Clarke, John Henry 1853–1931

The Edinburgh-trained emminent homoeopathic physician. Editor of the *Homoeopathic World*, consultant at the Royal London Homoeopathic Hospital; president of the international congress (1906), Clarke made major contributions to the literature throughout his life. His output was prolific and many of his writings, particularly his *Dictionary of Practical Materia*

Medica is standard reference to date.
Major writings are:
1885 *Prescriber*
1890 *Dictionary of Domestic Medicine*
1892 *Rheumatism and Sciatica*
1893 *Therapeutics of Serpent Poisons*
1894 *Diseases of Glands and Bones*
1895 *Diseases of Heart and Arteries*
1896 *Heart Repertory*
1900 *Dictionary of Practical Materia Medica*
1904 *Clinical Repertory*
1904 *Life and Work of James Compton Burnett*
1905 *Homoeopathy Explained*
1906 *Whooping Cough, cured with Pertussis*
1907 *Thomas Skinner M.D.*
1908 *Radium as an internal Remedy*
1909 *Vital Economy*
1915 *Gunpowder as a war remedy*
1923 *Hahnemann and Paracelsus*
1925 *Constitutional Medicine*
1928 *Colds, hay-fever and Influenza*
      Indigestion its causes and cure.

Claustrophobia

A psychological problem that may be acute or long-standing.
There is considerable underlying insecurity coming to the surface
as irrational fears of confined spaces — especially of being shut-in
any tangible enclosed space or psychological situation where
there is any obstacle to easy retreat. There is profound fear of
fainting, or diarrhoea, collapse, weakness or nervous breakdown
or 'making a show'. Any sort of exhibition or drawing attention is
feared, yet often an underlying tendency at the same time.
REMEDIES
Arg. Nit, Lachesis, Aconitum, Ignatia, Natrum Mur.

Close, Stuart, M.D. (1860–1929)

The American homoeopath, professor of homoeopathic
philosophy at the New York homoeopathic medical college
1901–13.

Major writings include:
The Genius of Homoeopathy
1924 *Lectures and Essays on Homoeopathic Philosophy*

Coccalgia

Pain in the coccyx, or 'tail' of the vertebral cord. The symptoms may be constant or intermittent, and often follow a fall or trauma to the area. In others it is arthritic or sometimes of unknown origin.
REMEDIES
Rhus Tox, Ruta, Symphytum, Arnica.

Cocculus (Indian Cockle)

An important remedy for vertigo, nausea, dizzyness and light-headedness. Depression is a feature and generally all symptoms are worse at period times. Nausea of pregnancy, travel sickness, Paralysis of one limb. The periods are very painful and too early. A tendency to never stop talking and intolerence of tight-fitting clothing is often diagnostic.

Coffea Cruda (Coffee)

The remedy for restlessness, agitation and insomnia. Neuralgic pains are common — of the teeth or head. Palpitations with a rapid heart beat are common side effects of too much coffee drinking. Generally the mind is over-active, unable to relax, which creates much of the extreme sensitivity.

Coffee

Because coffee is an artificial stimulant and a plant poison acting on the cardiovascular and central nervous systems it is not generally recommended during homoeopathic treatment. The initial stimulant effect is quickly followed by one of tension and a 'strung out' effect followed by a 'low'. It is a drug of social addiction. During treatment intake should be avoided or lessened considerably as it tends to reduce the efficiency of the remedies. For many years it has been suspected as having a possible link with cancer formation, particularly of the pancreas — a tumour which has increased in frequency over the past twenty years. In the U.S. it has now been statistically linked with this type of cancer as a causative factor. Where there is a craving for coffee to an addictive degree with over-excitability, give *Coffea*. When also associated with irritability *Nux vom* is indicated.

Cold Sores

Localised infective areas of either upper or lower lip, associated with catarrh or the common cold. The cause is a localised viral infection of the Herpes Simplex type which is usually benign and clears up within a few days. Only in rare cases is there secondary infection and a boil or carbuncle develops.

REMEDIES

Pulsatilla 6 for cold sores of the upper lip.

Natrum Mur 6 for cold sores affecting the lower lip area.

Colic

There is severe abdominal pain which causes doubling-up in an attempt to find relief. The pain is caused by spasm of smooth muscle because of irritation provoked by infection — especially the common intestinal colic. A stone may provoke renal colic or gall-bladder colic. The condition is relieved by heat and rest, although at times there may be considerable agitation and restlessness. When severe and due to the passage of a stone in the bile or ureteric passages, there is pallor, collapse and shock due to the severity of the pain.

REMEDIES

Colocynth for renal colic with shock.

Mag. phos for intestinal colic.

Chelidon for biliary colic.

Arnica for shock.

Colitis

This is an increasingly and potentially dangerous condition, now seen at all ages from childhood onwards. There is inflammation and sometimes ulceration of the lining mucosal layer of the descending large bowel or colon, with the passage of fresh blood, mucous and diarrhoea. The whole of the area is inflamed and irritated — the cause unknown. In many cases there is an underlying stress factor present with typical 'bottling up' of all feelings, particularly anger or rage, a tendency to be of rigid obsessional make-up, where everything is unhealthily pushed-down and denied. Hospitalisation and surgery is needed for severe cases, although an operation can often be avoided by the correct homoeopathic approach.

REMEDIES

Natrum Mur, China, Arsenicum, Phosphorus, Podophyllum, Phosphoric Acid.

The Common Cold (coryza)

The common condition of acute viral infection, common in all ages, particularly in the winter months. There is an acute sore throat, nasal congestion, headache, cough, mild temperature and general malaise. Mild depression and exhaustion may follow the attack. The usual precipitating causes are cold, damp, fatigue and especially some form of psychological stress undermining vitality and resistance.

REMEDIES

Arsenicum Alb in the 30c potency taken hourly when there is marked debility and weakness with exhaustion, burning pains, headache and diarrhoea.

Nux. Vom. 30c Where the appetite is affected with constipation, nausea and irritability.

Complaints (of the patient)

Complaints or symptoms are what the patient feels and experiences of their illness. This dis-ease is the key to homoeopathic prescribing and the basis of its individuality and accuracy. The complaints are listed and systemised in the Repertory, the most complete being Kent's Repertory which is a major reference volume linking symptoms, aggravations and ameliorating factors with individual remedies. It is very important that the patient reports every complaint however odd, bizarre or trivial to his doctor.

Complications of Homoeopathic Treatment

There are no true complication of homoeopathy except those reactions which are part of cure. They may appear abruptly as an aggravation of a previous state with apparent worsening of symptoms. This happens as the remedy 'gets hold' of the problem and makes it more available to the process of cure. When an earlier illness has been suppressed or not properly treated, then these former symptoms may reappear. Normally this is only temporary and a short-lived phase of the treatment.

Concepts of Homoeopathy

These are based on the Law of Similarities or 'Similar Similibus Curentur'. Let that which can provoke illness also cure it, or let like be treated by like. Use of the 'similar' remedy is the cornerstone of homoeopathy, matching the proving symptoms of the remedy or its known toxicology patterns to those of the patient. It is fundamental to homoeopathy that the single remedy is used in the highest potency whenever possible and that the remedy is not repeated as long as there is an improvement. Individualisation is prescribing for the individual patient and his symptoms rather than for a disease-pattern and is fundamental to the whole homoeopathic approach.

Confusion (mental)

The mental processes of clarity of thought, judgement and perception are clouded. The causes include infection with an associated high temperature, organic brain disease, arteriosclerosis, senility or psychological factors. Each must be clearly differentiated when diagnosis is made.
REMEDIES
Opium, Aconite, Natrum Mur, Cann. Sat, Sulph, Stramonium.

Conium Maculatum (Hemlock)

An ancient remedy used in homoeopathy for chronic lymphatic and glandular conditions, especially where there is fibrosis and hardening of the glands affected. The action is a very generalised one throughout the body but especially it has action on the uterus with spasm, painful scanty periods and on breast tissue with hardness and painless enlargement (*Bryonia*).

Conjunctivitis

Inflammation of the conjunctiva of the eye with redness, irritation, lachrymation and discomfort. Causes are local

irritation, infection, a foreign body — an eyelash is a common
one.

REMEDIES

Sulphur, Pulsatilla, Euphrasia in the 6th potency and as a local
eyebath using one drop of the mother tincture in the eye-wash
gives soothing relief.

Constipation

There is lack or absence of the usual bowel motion. Often the
cause is due to faulty bowel-habit and training, a poor diet lacking
in roughage, lack of exercise, refined food and the use of laxatives
over years so that natural tone is completely lost. When present,
most people quickly become over-anxious and do not give the
bowel enough time to respond before rushing back to yet another
laxative.

REMEDIES

Alumina when there is hardly any bowel action at all and where
aluminium pans have been used for a long period.

Nux. Vom. is indicated when there is desire but no push or ability
to expel the stool.

Bryonia is valuable when there is absence of desire and the stools
are small, dried and round, like sheep droppings.

Opium is recommended for severe and absolute constipation
without desire. In all cases take added bran with breakfast
commencing with a teaspoonful daily.

Constitutional prescribing

The homoeopathic remedy, usually given in high potency usually
which matches the temperament and physiological
configurations of the individual. When correctly prescribed it
stimulates a vital healing reaction and a liberating feeling of relief
and well-being. A recurrent problem is often resolved by the
'constitutional'. It is one of the most important principles of
homoeopathic prescribing.

Consultation guidelines for the patient

Relate all symptoms felt which cause complaint or discomfort —
however trivial. Do not give the diagnosis or supposed one unless
it is one feared or specifically asked for. Give every detail of the

problem including the time of onset and any known causes. Describe if the illness has occurred before at any time and if so when and how. Describe the progress of the illness, any new or recent symptoms, why you have come to see the doctor now and whether any homoeopathic remedies have been taken and their results. Describe any factors which either ameliorate or aggravate the condition with details of previous medical treatments or operations, including antibiotics or steroids. Mention any factors which have caused a change in the subsequent pattern of the disease. Give details of family or hereditary diseases known, especially T.B., cancer, diabetes. Try to give a general historical picture from birth onwards, with special areas of sensitivity or problem. Be natural and spontaneous with your doctor. If you are feeling anxious or uncomfortable — tell him at the time.

Convalescent Remedies

During this period it is important to remember that reserves of vitality are inevitably low, and that excessive fatigue or effort should be avoided — particularly during the early weeks.

Often there is a relapse after strain during this time which should be one of the quiet calm and consolidating of reserves.

REMEDIES

Arnica for post-operative convalescence three times daily, 6th potency.

Cadmium Phos. for after 'flu weakness and debility.

Kali Phos for weakness and lack of reserve after any illness.

China is indicated for more severe weakness and exhaustion after a long, drawn-out and debilitating illness.

Ferr. Met. when anaemia and pallor with shortness of breath is associated.

Staphysagria, for the immediate period after surgery.

Phytolacca Berry can be a useful tonic in mother tincture after illness.

Cough

There is irritation of the upper respiratory tract from a variety of causes. These vary from the common cold to bronchitis, laryngitis, polyps, substernal goitre. The cough may be dry or moist depending upon the condition of the mucosal lining. A further common cause and one not to be forgotten is the long-standing dry 'nervous' cough which is familiar and gives a degree of comfort to any new or unfamiliar settings.

REMEDIES

Bryonia — Dry cough.

Ipecacuanha — moist cough, rattling and loud.

Merc. Sol. — with yellow, infected phlegm.

Sulphur — if there is severe infection and pus formation.

Hydrastis — When the phleghm is thick and ropey.

Spongia — For an irritating, dry cough.

Pertussin — When the cough causes retching or nausea.

Natrum Sulph. — When associated with bronchitis and shortness of breath.

Drosera — Where a cough is dry, explosive and repetitive.

Natrum Mur — for a dry 'nervous' cough.

Cowperthwaite, Allen C, M.D. (1848–

The early American homoeopath, born in New Jersey and graduate of the Hahnemann college of homoeopathy, Philadelphia in 1869. For most of his life he practised in Illinois where he became editor of the *North-Western Journal of Homoeopathy* (1889–91). Professor of materia medica and diseases of women in the university of Iowa, he was also president of the American Institute of Homoeopathy. Poet and author as well as a physician, his major homoeopathic writings include:

1877 *Science in therapeutics.*
1880 *Elementary text-book of materia medica*
1882 *Text-book of materia medica.*
1888 *Disorders of Menstruation.*
1891 *Textbook of materia medica and therapeutics.*
Textbook of Gynaecology.

Cramps (nocturnal)

These usually occur in the calves or sometimes the dorsum of the feet. The cause is unknown but most probably they are circulatory in origin.

REMEDIES

Cuprum Arsenicum 6 is one of the most useful remedies, *Arsenicum* is indicated when they occur in the early hours — just after midnight and have a burning quality to them.

Kali Carb 6 is of value when cramps wake from sleep at a later

51

time, between 3–5 a.m.
Pulsatilla is indicated when brought on by the heat of the bed.

Crataegus (Hawthorn Berry)

The valuable heart tonic, usually prescribed as mother tincture to be taken in water. Main indications are palpitations, irregularity of beat, blood pressure, breathless on exertion, heart failure, sweating. Mentals-exhausted, flat, irritable.

Cravings for foods

These are often a manifestation of addiction to certain foods and are important because they give the clue to remedies, e.g. chocolate-craving — *Lycopodium*; Salt — *Natrum Mur*; fats, — *Sulphur*.

Croton Tiglium (Croton oil seeds)

The most extreme intestinal irritation with colic and explosive watery diarrhoea is characteristic. There is also severe skin irritation with burning eczema, or inflammation, the area bright red and burning (*Belladonna*).

Crystallography

Using patterns of crystallisation, it is now possible to clearly differenetiate mother tinctures of the remedies. Research in this area is giving encouraging results and it is hoped that physical differentiation of the individual spectrum-potencies will follow as techniques improve.

Cullen, Prof. William (1710–   )

The emminent eighteenth century physician who advocated treating the patient with the single remedy at a time when multiple prescribing or poly-pharmacy was particularly in vogue. His best known work was a treatise of *Materia Medica* published in 1790. When Hahnemann was translating this work into German he found himself in total disagreement with Cullen on the gastric action of China or Quinine in the treatment of Malaria. Because it was also a gastric bitter and tonic, this lead Cullen to recommend strychnine for the same condition. From this basic disagreement Hahnemann began taking Cinchona bark or quinine as a clinical experiment, quickly developing all the clinical symptoms of malaria and the first 'proving'.

Cuprum Aceticum (Copper Acetate)

One of the best remedies for cramps in the calves at night or spasms of colicy pains in the abdomen at night. Nocturnal asthma, hay fever. There are many chronic skin problems and the remedy is indicated in psoriasis.

Cuprum Arsenicosum (Arsenite of Copper)

A powerful remedy for chronic renal failure and uraemia. There are many burning neuralgic pains coupled with chillyness and cramping pains. Intense cold is a feature of the remedy with sweating, asthma or colic. Carbuncle.

Cure

For a true cure to occur there must be not just freedom from symptoms and relief from illness or pathology but also a freeing and liberation of the basic vital energy of the person. Freedom from abnormal and crippling exhaustion and fatigue with no reserves, the patient constantly tired and 'run down'. In addition, for a homoeopathic cure to occur there should have been some basic alteration in the patients disposition, attitudes and to a certain extent their perspectives and aims, especially when these have been previously blocked-off or vague, clouded and distorted so that the approach to living and to others was doomed to failure. In the highest potencies the remedies can correct this level of individual perception together with a freeing of vital energy to complete the cure. Just freedom from symptoms without the change of perception and perspective leaves a risk of further relapses.

Cystitis

There is infection of the bladder with symptoms of frequent desire to pass water, burning pain and often urgency. The urine may be cloudy or strong-smelling.

Cantharis, Causticum, Hepar Sulph, Sulphur Pyrogen, or *Terebinthina, Sabadilla.*

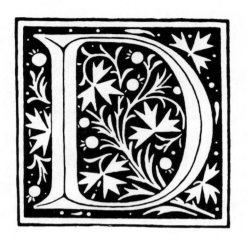

Dangers of Homoeopathy

These are in general rare and uncommon and when properly prescribed, homoeopathy is safe, non-toxic, non-addictive and does not cause psychological dependency. It is basic to homoeopathy that as soon as there is improvement, the remedy should be stopped. If remedies are continued needlessly during the period of recovery, they can in some cases stimulate the re-appearance of the original symptoms and make them chronic. Such ill-advised prescribing is not in keeping with homoeopathic principles. There is another area of caution concerning the remedy *Silicea* which is very deep acting and a powerful treatment of encysted conditions. It should be used with caution and only in low potency when there is a history of old T.B. to avoid any risk of a cyst being re-activated into renewed activity by stimulating the breakdown of scar-tissue and drainage of any residual old infection or pus. Such caution evidences the importance of a thorough knowledge of homoeopathic principles and past medical history of every patient.

Dead Fingers

The common problem where the ends of the fingers become white and bloodless due to poor circulatory control. It is often familial and may occur equally in summer as well as winter, although it is always aggravated by cold. The condition is not usually dangerous to health unless very severe when tissue-damage and ulceration may occur. The latter is rare however (Raynaud's disease).

REMEDIES

Silicea 6, Hammamelis. Where *Silicea* is not sufficient to stimulate a response, sometimes *Carbo Veg* or *Agaricus* are required.

Decalcification

A general condition whereby bones become transparent and more brittle causing osteoporosis or thinning of bone structure on x-ray examination. Major causes are aging with disuse of joints. An excessive intake of certain vitamins without caution over a long period may also cause calcium to be removed from bones and sometimes laid-down in other tissues to form a calculus. Trauma or infection, especially T.B. or osteomyelitis are other causes.

REMEDIES

Calc. Carb., Calc. Fluor.

Definition of Homoeopathy

Homoeopathy comes from the two Greek words *Homeos*, meaning equal or like and *Pathos* which is suffering or anguish. The basis of all homoeopathy is treatment using remedies which in their unprepared and often toxic state, cause similar symptoms to those of the patient. Homoeopathy is a uniquely individual treatment using natural substances in their vitalised form, prepared by a process of dilution to stimulate the natural curative energies inherent within each individual. Increasing the dilution of the remedy-substance — although lessening its actual material content, paradoxically increases the strength and power of the remedy-substance and deepens its action. The remedy must be well-prescribed however to be effective and match the overall picture of individual symptoms. The correct remedy is called the simillimum and is the underlying principle of *Similia Similibus Curentur* given to us by Paracelsus. The Latin inscription is best translated as 'let like be treated by like' — the homoeopathic cornerstone and major treatment principle.

Delirium

The state of mental confusion, over-activity and hyper-excitability usually associated with a high temperature or toxic state. There is wild delusional anxiety, disorientation, fear and restless, sometimes violent behaviour.

REMEDIES

Belladonna, Croton Tig, Hyoscyamus and *Stramonium.*

Depression

The familiar state of diminished spirits, with flatness, sadness, disinterest and lack of energy. Various physical symptoms may be associated, for example chronic back pain or exhaustion — in fact any complaint that is not responding to treatment and is recurrent may hide a depressive illness. The causes are many and varied, but include a physical shock to the system as miscarriage, childbirth, 'flu, glandular fever. In most cases there is an underlying psychological cause — either recent or remote, which was traumatic and led to feelings of sadness or failure. Mourning and loss are well-known factors in depression and these can often recur, triggered-off by any event that floods the person with feelings, often denied at the time.

REMEDIES

Aurum Met, Ignatia, Sepia, Natrum Mur, Gelesemium, Pulsatilla, Lycopodium, Arg. Nit.

Dewey, W.A., M.D. (1858–1938)

The emminent American homoeopath, professor emeritus of materia medica and therapeutics, University of Michegan. Major writings are:

Essentials of Homoeopathic Materia Medica
Essentials of Homoeopathic Therapeutics
The Twelve Tissue Remedies (1934), co-author.

Diagnosis by the homoeopathic physician

This is always made on the totality of symptoms and according to the individual's response to underlying causative factors and their effect on intrinsic vital energy reserves. Diagnosis is made according to the remedy indicated by the overall pattern of symptoms rather than any underlying pathology, which the homoeopath considers of secondary importance to primary undermining of reserves and vitality. Accordingly a problem strictly in homoepathy is not named as 'arthritis' or 'sinusitis', but rather according to the indicated remedy, for example *Rhus Tox* or *Pulsatilla*.

Diarrhoea

Excessive and uncontrollable looseness of normal bowel action. Causes are usually infection, but it may be emotional in some cases or associated with underlying constipation which is the real problem.

REMEDIES

Aconite when the diarrhoea is sudden and acute — the patient extremely restless and apprehensive.

Arsenicum, the stool watery, the patient prostrated yet restless and anxious.

China for attacks of watery-green stools as with infantile diarrhoea or food poisoning.

Sulphur is indicated where the stools are offensive, green and slimey.

Podophyllum is a useful remedy when there are watery-yellow painless stools.

Veratrum Alb. is for diarrhoea where the patient is collapsing, the stools painful, watery, with nausea, vomiting, weakness and profuse sweating.

Diet during Homeopathic treatment

Extremes in any form should be avoided in order that vital energy be given maximum chance to recover and not wasted before being fully re-established with resistance and resources strong. Diet should therefore be regular, light and simple, avoiding excessive spices, flavouring or rich food. The intake of tobacco should be kept to a minimum as also coffee and tea — both really best avoided altogether during treatment. Foods should be steamed or lightly cooked and no added vitamins taken. The contraceptive pill should be continued as before but any previous side-effects carefully noted. In general during treatment, try to avoid instant frozen foods wherever possible, also those containing sodium glutamate, colorants or preservative of the supermarket-convenience type. Eat fresh but not over-cooked dishes during the period of the remedy's action. High-fibre, raw foods are often helpful, supporting the eliminating function of toxic matters and regular bowel movement.

Digitalis (Foxglove)

Tincture of the leaves of the mature plant. Indications are collapse, with a slow weak pulse, palpitations, angina, pneumonia, asthma and urinary infection. Depression is common. They want to be alone. Also prostate problems, liver congestion with nausea, lack of appetite.

Dilatation of the Stomach

There is distention with pain and discomfort of the upper abdomen and stomach region or epigastrium.

REMEDIES

Carbo Veg where most of the trouble is in the upper abdomen and stomach area.

Lycopodium indicated when symptoms are situated somewhat lower down in the abdomen.

Arg. Nit. useful for more general flatulence and distention particularly whenever there is great intolerance of heat or an airless atmosphere.

Dilution of the remedies

This is the uniquely homoeopathic way of diluting the remedies. Using the centisimal scale most frequently and succussing or violently agitating the dilutant each time it is 'reduced' in content at each stage of the preparation although the potency or strength of action is paradoxically increased. Succussing gives the remedy its unique homoeopathic properties and differentitates the remedy from a simple vaccine formed by dilution without dynamitisation. The remedies may also be dilted on the millinesimal scale of one drop in a thousand dilutent fluid up to thousandth dilution or M.M. potency using a machine designed to automatically make up the higher potencies. In general the lower dilutions of 6c act purely at a tissue level and only the higher potencies act on the mentals or psychological processes as well as the tissues and much more constitutionally. But whatever the dilution, it is fundamental not to repeat the dosage or potency once there has been an improvement and positive response.

Dioscorea Villosa (the Wild Yam)

Tincture of the fresh root, first proved by Burt. Indicated for severe colicky pains of the stomach and bowel. Biliary colic. Restless. Pregnancy morning sickness. A remedy for severe pain, particularly of a colicy neuralgic type. The main areas affected are the abdomen and bowel with sudden bouts of colic and flatulence, better for movement. Early morning diarrhoea (*Sulphur*).

Disease

For the homoeopath, disease is not seen so much in terms of invasion or infection but rather in terms of primary dis-functioning or dis-ease which was fundamental in originally undermining the healthy process of vitality and resistance. Invasion or infection with loss of functioning is seen as a much later secondary phenomena. In origin, dis-ease is usually either psychological or inherited due to the presence of an underlying miasm or familiar factor constantly undermining vitality. Stress is the commonest of all present-day disease factors leading to weakness and increased susceptibility to all illness from the common cold to a heart-attack.

Dosage

This is often an area of confusion to many. But dosage is not so important initially and only requires attention at a later date when considering the level and depth of the primary causative disturbance. What matters most is that the remedy be prescribed on sound homoeopathic principles according to the law of similitudes and not repeated once there has been a response. Certainly in the problem of chronic recurrent disease, higher potencies are often the only answer, sometimes in the 200 or 10M strength or higher. The remedy will act in any potency or strength for the well-being of the patient so that accuracy of remedy is the priority and dosage a secondary consideration, though nevertheless an important one for the physician.

Drosera Rotundifolia (Sundew)

Tincture of the whole plant. Its main action is on the upper respiratory tract with a recurrent barking type of cough, nausea and vomiting, Whooping cough. All symptoms are worse in bed, after midnight and from warmth. It has a role in the prophylaxis of T.B.

Drugs

Drugs are largely synthetic preparations used by the allopath in an attempt to block or suppress the natural process of illness patterns. The priority is always the alleviation of symptoms. Even the natural drugs of plant origin, such as digitalis are now prepared synthetically and their naturally occuring alkaloids and other active principles are lost to the patient in favour of more 'scientific' and convenient ones. The homoeopath will always put the needs of the patient before blanket-principles. Where a drug is required he will prescribe it, but in general he considers that most drugs are over-prescribed and suppress rather than stimulate a healthy response to the underlying condition — which is the true and real cause of the patient's malaise. In general no form of suppression is used by the homoeopath unless pain or suffering is unbearable. A gentle stimulation of the fundamental well-being of the individual is the aim and powerful artificial remedies often oppose these fundamental principles.

Drysdale, John, M.D. (-   )

The Edinburgh graduate, and friend of Simpson, who settled in Liverpool and founded the Liverpool dispensary in 1837. There was a severe cholera outbreak in the city in 1849. As with the similar London outbreak, the results with homoeopathic treatment were outstanding, well below the corresponding allopathic figures with only 25.7% mortality. As a result of these statistics he was invited to apply for the post of physician to the city's childrens hopsital, but opposition was so considerable that he was forced to eventually withdraw. Co-editor of the *British Journal of Homoeopathy*.

Dulcamara (Woody Nightshade)

Prepared from fresh stems and leaves just before flowering. The 'barometer of remedies' with aggravation of all symptoms from any change of weather but especially worse for cold or damp. Indicated for throat or chest infections, nasal catarrh, warts, hay fever, laryngitis with complete loss of voice. Summer diarrhoea.

63

Dunham, Carroll. M. D. (1828–1877)

The distinguished New York homoeopath. Qualifying in 1850, like Boenninghausen, he was converted to the homoeopathic approach following a dramatic personal cure when conventional methods had failed. A pupil of Constantine Hering in Philadelphia, he also worked with Boenninghausen in Munster. An early advocate of the single remedy and if possible the single dose, he became president of the National Homoeopathic Institute in 1876. Translator of Boenninghausen and author of numerous review articles, he was editor of the *American Homoeopathic Review*.

Dynamics of cure

This is the intrinsic energy of the patient, lost to him by the underlying illness and a direct result of the true basic disease which lies beneath the obvious presenting complaints and symptoms. Homoeopathy is dynamic because well-chosen potentised remedies have sufficient energy within them, enhanced by the dilution process to overcome many of these blocks which shut-away and bind the patient's individual and ultimate vitality. Freeing the energy of the patient by the intrinsic power of the remedy makes for dynamic medicine and a dynamic cure.

Dysentery

Acute bacterial infective disease of the bowel, endemic in certain countries and marked by high temperature, collapse, pain, the passage of watery diarrhoea, blood and mucous. It is especially dangerous to infants and the elderly.

REMEDIES

Aconite, Arsenicum also *Sulphur* for chronic cases. *Mercurius 6* for the acute symptoms, *Nux Vom* and *Colocynth* for severe cramps. When the case is at all severe hospitalisation is required when available.

Dysmenorrhoea

The periods are painful and often irregular.

REMEDIES

Pulsatilla for variable pains, tearfulness and intolerance of heat.

Frequency of urination may be present.

Nux. Vom. where there is nausea, upset digestive functioning and irritability.

Chamomilla where the pains are severe, worse in the lower abdomen with irritability.

Caulophyllum where there are writhing generalised pains in abdomen and back.

Sepia where the pains are very low down in the abdomen and have a dragging-down quality.

Veratrum for menstrual colic with prostration where bed-rest is essential during the spasms.

Dyspepsia

The common problem of indigestion — most commonly due to over-indulgence or eating too quickly. Allergy or infection are other causes. Symptoms are pain, flatulence a sense of fullness and malaise, with acidity.

REMEDIES

Nux. Vom., Carbo Veg., Sulphur.

Dyspnoea

Difficulty and shortage of breath, either at rest or on the very least effort. The causes are many but most commonly it is associated with either asthma, chronic emphysema, bronchitis, infection as pneumonia, collapse of the lung, or as an aspect of cardiac malfunctioning with oedema of the lungs.

REMEDIES

For Asthma, *Phosphorus, Medorrhinum, Arsenicum, Kali Carb.* *Bronchitis – Natrum Sulph.* Where there is collapse with oedema give *Ant. Tart, Arnica* or *Veratrum Alb.* Where there is sudden collapse of lung (pneumothorax) give *Arnica, Aconite, Phosphorus* according to symptoms and hospitalise.

Dys. Co. (Bach)

The bowel nosode. Not related to previous attacks of dysentery. There is typical marked anticipatory nervous tension with lack of confidence. Psychological symptoms are particularly marked with phobias, as claustrophobia. The build is thin with fair hair and love of fatty foods. Hay fever, blinding headaches, chronic diarrhoea, frequent colds particularly with the phobic mental component. Chronic indigestion, distention, duodenal ulcer, discomfort after meals.

Dysuria

The condition of difficulty or hesitancy in passing water. It is often commoner in men but may occur in either sex. The commonest causes are due to enalrged prostate, infection, post-operative nerve-bruising or after childbirth. I have also seen it following lumbar-puncture and catherisation in women. Remedies for prostate disease include *Sabal Serrulata 6.* Where the problem is infective give either *Hepar Sulph* or *Cantharis, Causticum* or *Merc. Sol,* according to the indications and symptoms. When the problem is post-operative or after delivery give *Causticum 6.* There are some cases when the problem is purely nervous in origin and in these cases *Natrum Mur* is the remedy in high potency of at least 200c.

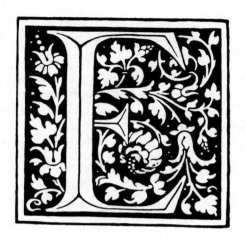

Ear Ache

Usually due to infection of either the outer chamber of the ear (external otitis) or most commonly to middle ear disease (otitis media). It is extremely painful, with high temperatures and agitation.

REMEDIES

Aconite in the acute and immediately painful phase.
Belladonna where there is heat, red face, and high fever.
Sulphur for chronic recurrent cases.
Pulsatilla where the pain is variable and intermittent, worse for warmth or heat.
Mercurius 6 when there is discharge.

Early Diagnosis (importance of)

In all cases of illness, as soon as diagnosis can be made and treatment started, the better. In homoeopathy — as with any form of treatment once a problem becomes chronic, or long-standing it takes longer to heal because vital energies have become exhausted, the energy-reaction to cure is slow to respond and takes longer. For example when a problem of psoriasis or even simple eczema is treated at the early stages, response is usually immediate. But after several months, or years, following innumerable failures of treatment, both vital energy is exhausted as well as the patient psychologically, and time must elapse before a healing-reaction occurs.

Eating-out, fear of

This is a common psychological condition with underlying lack of confidence which has become polarised to the area of putting food or drink into the mouth. The usual symptom is one of tension when handling a cup or glass and there is anxiety about drawing attention to handshaking and tremor. It can occur at any age and may only be of passing significance, although sometimes long-standing and present over many years. There may be other phobic anxieties also present and associated as claustrophobia, fear of crowds or being shut-into any situation without an obvious or easy exit.

REMEDIES
Arg. Nit, Ignatia, Lycopodium, Pulsatilla, Sulphur.

Eczema

The common chronic skin ailment of infants and adults sometimes occurring from the very earliest weeks of life. It is not advisable to suppress the condition using steroid ointments as is the fashion — from the youngest baby onwards. This creates a more chronic condition just under the skin with little or no symptom-relief. The exact cause is usually not known but there are often strong familial tendencies to the condition and it is quite common to see one of the parents with the same or similar condition as the child. Commonest symptoms are redness and a slightly raised irritation sometimes with cracks, oozing or bleeding, around the flexure areas of the limbs, wrists and hands. In severe cases, the whole of a limb can be swollen, the eczema bleeding from scratching, the areas bandaged-up or stuck to the stockings, and the child stiff with swelling, unable to sit down and crying with pain. There may be considerable flaking of the skin areas which falls like snow on the carpet of the consulting room.

REMEDIES
Sulphur, Petroleum, Apis, Graphites, Belladonna, Rhus Tox.

Emotional Problems

The homoeopathic treatment of emotional problems is in general very efficient giving an early feeling of well-being and confidence to the patient that allows him to better perceive both his own feelings and motivations as well as those of others in the

70

psychological environment. All major remedies contain an emotional sphere of action in their make-up and this can be used to the advantage of the patient who comes for treatment. Some remedies have these emotional or mental areas of activity particularly emphasised and these include *Natrum Mur, Ignatia, Pulsatilla, Lycopodium, Arg. Nit., Phosphorus, Sulph.*

Emphysema

The common and chronic chest infection, often the aftermath of chronic bronchitis. The chest is large, fixed and barrel-shaped, with breathing shallow and limited. The patient is quickly short of breath on effort, and liable to attacks of winter bronchitis.
REMEDIES
Natrum Sulph, Arsenicum, Phosphorus, Ant. Tart., Hepar Sulph., Spongia, Tub. Bov, Sulphur.

Epilepsy

The recurrent illness with fits or convulsions, either severe as a major attack 'grand mal' with loss of consciousness and bladder control, or the minor, 'petit mal' form with temporary lapses of consciousness and awareness. The cause is usually of unknown origin although in some cases there has been trauma or infection in the past which has quite clearly preceded the onset. In general the treatment should be in the hands of an experienced physician. It often happens that the patient has warning or an aura, of an imminent attack and they can sometimes be prevented at this stage or take precautions to minimise danger to themselves or others.
REMEDIES
Belladonna, Aconite, Sulphur, Arnica.

Equisetum (Scouring Bush)

Tincture of the whole fresh plant. Mainly indicated for bladder infection with typical irritation, constant frequency and cystitis, passing small amounts of urine. Pain in the bladder and kidney region. Bed-wetting. The bladder feels incompletely empty after passing urine.

Errors of prescribing

These are less important in homoeopathy than in other treatments because there are no side-effects of the homoeopathic remedy and usually the wrong remedy simply fails to act or elicite a response in the patient. It sometimes happens that the patient is sensitive to a particular remedy which gives a very active response — in itself neither a danger nor undesirable, but it may cause anxiety, so that the remedy is best avoided in future treatments. This is often the result of previous suppressant treatments, rather than a fault of the remedy itself. When this happens any remedy can quite simply be antidoted by its opposite or neutralised by giving *Sulphur 6* three times daily until the reaction passes.

Euonymus Europea (Spindle Tree)

Tincture of the fresh seed. Indicated for severe diarrhoea, cutting abdominal pains, chest pain with collapse, angina. It is essentially a left-sided remedy.

Eupatorium Purpureum (Trumpet Weed, Gravel Root)

Tincture of the root. Useful in bladder problems, incontinence, impotency, prostatic problems, bladder irritation, uterine weakness, sterility. Primarily a left-sided remedy. All symptoms are aggravated by movement.

Euphrasia Officinalis (Eye Bright)

Tincture of the whole plant. Mainly an eye remedy especially for conjunctivitis, inflammation, lachrymation, swelling of the lower eyelid, pain, intolerance of light. Also hay fever and measles. Useful in congestion of the prostate. Yawning in the open air. Fatigue and insomnia is characteristic.

Examination of the Patient

This is an essential part of homoeopathic procedure in order to make a diagnosis at every level for the patient's well-being. In homoeopathy the patient is an individual and this comes before all other considerations including those of homoeopathic principles. Where there is a mechanical problem, this needs to be corrected — narrowing due to scar-tissue needs dilating before

72

homoeopathic treatment can work fully. This requires a physical examination to be certain that the case is one where homoeopathy is properly indicated and to avoid falling into the unrealistic trap of thinking that homoeopathy is a panacea for all illness. The need to exclude physical organic features is the major reason for making an examination in all cases. The homoeopathic doctor is foremost a physician and needs to look, touch, feel as well as listen — the fundamentals of all good doctoring.

Examinations — fear of

This is the common 'funk' situation whenever there is a threat of something new and unfamiliar with the possibility of failing to live up to high, often unrealistic standards. All of this makes for a conscience that is perfectionistic, rigid and intolerant of failure so that the examination situation — however important is nevertheless over-valued, made too significant and lacking an overall viewpoint, the person paralysed by fear of their own making. Homoeopathy is particularly effective in just this type of problem and can lead to a release of more confidence and balance when the prescription is right.
REMEDIES
Arg. Nit, Gelsemium, Aconitum, Lycopodium.

Excitement and Elation

There are a variety of causes for this, varying from simple healthy youth and exhilaration, to alcoholism, brain-damage, manic-depressive disease, drug-abuse or a high temperature. Most cases respond well to the indicated remedies which include *Belladona, Stramonium* and *Hyoscyamus.*

Exhaustion

This is a common problem, seen increasingly in the young. The causes may be a physical with underlying anaemia or chronic infection, sometimes the results of influenza, or one of the more chronic debilitating diseases as hepatitis or glandular fever. Often there is no obvious cause to be found and the patient is depressed because of their lack of energy. Not uncommonly the reason lies with the lifestyle, lack of adequate sleep, regular exercise and fresh air. There is no overall plan or rhythm, the body poisoned by over-refined instand convenience-foods which fail to give proper nourishment.

REMEDIES

Arsenicum for acute cases,

China following an illness such as 'flu,

Arnica is generally useful,

Kali Phos. will boost energy if the vital supplies are not completely exhausted,

Kali Carb may be indicated in cases where anxiety is marked.

But whatever remedy is given, the underlying cause must always be diagnosed and corrected.

Eye Problems

These vary enormously and respond well to the homoeopathic approach. Because the area is so specialised as well as delicate they are best treated by a physician with special experience in the area. The common problem of conjunctivitis responds well to *Sulphur* or *Euphrasia.* Styes often clear up with *Pulsatilla 6,* infection with *Mercurius 6.*

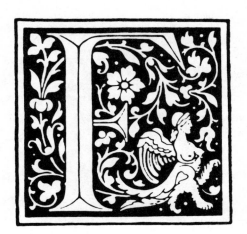

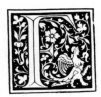

Faculty of Homoeopathy

The governing body of the homoeopathic physicians in the U.K., based at the Royal London Homoeopathic Hospital. Many of its members are on the staff of the hospital. It governs the teaching, training and membership examination of the physician for the post-graduate homoeopathic degree following general medical qualification. The faculty is responsible for standards of prctise in the country as well as for research, the publication of literature and information. It is linked with other countries and helps to organise national and international conferences representing the profession generally at all levels. The present secretary (1983) is Colonel M. Barraclough.

Failure to respond to the Homoeopathic treatment

There can be many reasons, but often it is because the patient is impatient and wants an immediate magical cure which just does not exist. It is certain that in some cases the response to homoeopathy can be rapid and dramatic, but this does not always happen and rapidity of response depends on many factors including the length of time a the problem has been present, the amount and type of previous treatments and whether they have been designed to suppress or limit vital responses. Also patients vary with the quality of their intrinsic Vital Energy, sometimes a response is undermined by long periods of stress or a nutrition which does not sustain it, lacking intrinsic vitality and an

77

'appearance' food only. Other factors are due to wrong prescribing — quite simply the correct remedy has not been given in the best potency for the particularly individual.

The remedy may be inactive, or inadvertently neutralised and therefore ineffective. In some cases there is an underlying mechanical problem or condition which creates a barrier to cure because of obstruction or perhaps a surgical or dental condition — as an abscess that cannot drain naturally. Such conditions must first be corrected by the most appropriate treatment before homoeopathy can give a positive reaction and thrust towards health. Chronic disease due to miasmic factors was long regarded by Hahnemann as a cause of poor response to treatment in certain cases and led to his theory of action of Miasms.

Particularly Psora can lead to a weak or absent response even where a remedy is well-indicated.

REMEDIES

Any underlying mechanical problem must be dealt with initially. Give *Sulphur* in the 30th potency, or the most appropriate Nosode.

Fainting

See Syncope

Falls — Cause and treatment of

These may be a simple accident of the inquisitive child from careless inattention or part of life's inevitable tumbles as a grown-up world is explored. In others they are part of general accident-proneness (see section), and need special treatment and attention. In the elderly a fall is always serious and can led to fractures and immobilisation for weeks or months — the cause due to poor vision, sudden dizzyness, or weakness of limbs and movement.

REMEDIES

Arnica for shock and bruising,

Bellis Perennis for tendon and muscle strain.

Rhus Tox for any strain,

Calcarea when due to weak ankles,

Kali Carb where there is a tendency to accident proneness,

Lycopodium for general clumsyness,

Ruta, when the vision is weak causing lack of awareness of obstacles.

Rhus Tox when the cause is one of slowness and rheumatism getting off balance or for any muscle strain.

78

Farrington, Ernest Albert. M.D. (1847–1885)

The emminent American homoeopath, physician and lecturer of the Hahnemann college, Philadelphia. Editor of Hahnemann's condensed *Materia medica.*
Writings include:
(1887) *A Clinical Material Medica.*

Fasting — dangers of

A mild and temporary fast with fruit or vegetable juices, diluted with 50% spring water has much to commend it provided that it is not continued more than two days and that it has been adequately prepared for by at least one day of raw foods. Similarly a fruit fast is also beneficial provided also that it has been thought about, and the system is not loaded with acid fruits which do not agree with the needs and constitution of the patient. A prolonged and more severe fast can sometimes also be both indicated and beneficial. In all cases it should only be undertaken under supervision and in conditions of rest and repose — in peaceful surroundings if possible. The major danger of a severe fast is that of combining it with exposure to heat, especially of mid-summer. It can then cause extreme weakness and exhaustion of the vital energies to a dangerous level and in one of my cases was clearly the cause of severe anginal attacks in a hitherto healthy young woman. The fasting was quite unindicated medically and prolonged to a dangerous degree. The causes of recurrent fasting is often obsessional and psychological with a distorted body image. See section on *Anorexia Nervosa.*

Fatigue

See Exhaustion.

Fear

Whenever fear is the predominant emotion which overwhelms a person the remedy indicated is *Aconitum.* This is helpful whenever any condition has been precipitated by fear, even where it has occurred many years before.

Feet — restless

Fidgety or restless feet is commonly seen in an overactive child, nervous adolescent or over-anxious elderly person, unable to relax. They tend to be always on the move, doing something, up-and-down, throughout the day.

REMEDIES
Zincum Met, Arsenicum, Rhus Tox.

Fever

The common condition of elevated temperature usually due to underlying infection. Bed-rest, fluids only — mainly fruit juices (grape or apple) are particularly appropriate, sponge down until the temperature subsides. The cause must be ascertained in all cases and treated.

REMEDIES
Belladonna, Phytolacca, Arsenicum, Aconitum.

Ferrum Metallicum (the metal Iron)

Trituration of the metal Iron. The principle indications are iron-deficiency anaemia with flushed cheeks, pallor, weakness, exhaustion, shortness of breath. There is irritability with the least exertion. Often allergic to eggs.

Ferrum Phosphoricum (Ferric Phosphate of Iron)

Developed by Schlüessler. Mainly indicated for recurrent coughs and colds with anaemia, bronchitis, recurrent middle ear infections, laryngitis, rheumatism.

Fibroids

This is the simple fibrous tumour of the uterus, seen increasingly in young women. The cause is unknown, but would appear to be due to hormonal imbalance, possibly of stress origin. When the fibroids are large causing pressure symptoms on the bladder, they are best dealt with surgically. In early cases, the fibroids small and not causing obstruction give *Conium Mac 6* three times daily.

Finke, Bernard, M.D. (-   )

The homoeopath who first developed the C M potency.

First Aid

Homoeopathy is one of the most effective forms of treatment for first-aid conditions of the home. Any bleeding must be stopped by local pressure, the wound cleaned with *Calendula* ointment or lotion. A foreign body must be removed — e.g. pirces of glass or splinters. If necessary hospitalise to remove a foreign body if this cannot be done in the home. Give *Arnica* for shock, *Aconitum 6* for shock where there is fear and restlessness. *Ledum 6* for small clean penetrating wounds. Where the wound is more red and swollen use *Apis 6*. If the area is red, hot and inflamed — *Belladonna 6*. When there is weakness from loss of blood give *China 6*. If the patient is shocked and collapsed, keep warm in a blanket, with plenty of hot drinks. Give *Veratrum Alb 6* when pale, cold and collapsing. In all cases, haemorrhage, and shock must be given priority treatment. Use the Bach rescue remedy for shock, 5 drops every 15 minutes, every 5 minutes if severe, *Arsenicum* for restlessness. *Hypericum* for lacerated wounds with pain shooting up the limb. If in doubt call a physician or hospitalise at once.

Fissure

In many ways this resembles a fistula, but the tract or passage into the tissues is blind and does not connect with any internal organ or bowel, so that there is no discharge, other than from the local inflammation.

The commonest site is often an anal fissure when a crack appears in the anal mucosal lining of the bowel, causing the most excruciating pain on bowel movement. There may be discharge of blood from the fissure onto the stools from the abrasion and irritation or it may result in constipation from fear of a bowel movement. The stool must be softened — either by taking bran or olive oil in the diet for a few days and *Calendula* ointment should be applied twice daily to the area affected.
REMEDIES
Silicea 6.

81

Fistula

This is frequently a chronic condition with an irritating discharge, sometimes infected from a tract which connects the skin or exterior of the body with one of the internal organs or alimentary tract. It may be artificial and intentional when carried out as part of a surgical procedure for drainage. When chronic the acute initial condition failed to heal for some reason. It may also be due to trauma or infection — the inflammation tracking down from an infected area to form a natural drainage point at the exterior. The latter is healthy and positive provided that the fistula heals and closes up subsequently and is not a constant cause of trouble and irritation.

REMEDIES

Calcarea and *Silicea*, but DOT NOT use *Silicea* when the fistula is the result of an old T.B. condition.

As long as a fistula is still actively draining a condition, it should never be interfered with or surgically removed and stitched up. This can drive a disease-process deeper and create a more serious condition. One patient had a discharging fistula-in-ano excised surgically and closed. A year later she developed breast cancer! The link is not absolute or provable statistically, but the suspicion is there sufficently strongly not to interfere with what nature has provided. Drainage and free-flow of discharges from the body must in all cases be allowed to occur without obstruction whenever they occur. An emminent colleague reported another case of breast cancer which followed a woman changing from vaginal menstrual pads to internal tampons — only a few months prior to the lump being present. I am not of course putting this forward as a cause of breast cancer, but I am emphasising the importance of not obstructing the passage of natural flows from the body whether periodic or otherwise. In all cases irritation and blockage by synthetic material which does not suit the system is never recommended and as much care should go into the size and choice of tampons as with anything else to do with the care and healthy functioning of the body.

Flatulence

The sensation of being bloated or over-full in the upper abdominal or epigastric area, sometimes also felt in the chest. It may be due to the habit of aerophagy or swallowing air. Commonly seen in children and sometimes adults. Flatulence is also provoked by indigestion, rapid, hurried meals, not chewed or digested and where there is underlying stress.

REMEDIES

Carbo Veg, Nux Vom, Sulpur, Lycopodium, Arg. Nit.

Fleury, Rudoph, M.D. (–)

The emminent contemporary Swiss homoeopath. Graduate of Zurich. Having studied in Paris and Vienna he settled in Berne to establish his practise there. President of the Swiss Homoeopathic Society since 1950, and member of the International league since 1916. Especially reknown for having introduced new methods in case-taking. Editor of the *World Directory of Homoeopathic Physicians* (1967).

'Flu

The common epidemic influenzal condition which can occur at any time of year and in any age-group. The symptoms are usually high temperature, prostration, aching pains in the limbs and joints, loss of appetite, sore throat, constipation, sometimes diarrhoea, depression. Treatment must include bed-rest during the febrile period and fruit-juices only followed by a light, easily digestible diet. The condition is particularly dangerous to the elderly when great care must be taken to avoid chest complications from premature exposure to cold or chill afterwards. For the very frail and elderly, antibiotics are often advisable with homoeopathy in a secondary supportive role.

REMEDIES

Consider the specific influenzal nosode, *Aconitum, Arsenicum, Nux. Vom. Cadmium Phos* or *Kali Phos* during the convalescent period.

Fluoric Acid (Hydro-fluoric Acid)

Prepared from Calcium Fluoride and Sulphuric Acid. A remedy for chronic infections, acting on bone and scar tissue with a tendency to the formation of local infective areas. Whitlow, fistula, ulcers of the skin, varicose ulcers, fall within its range.

Food Poisoning

Acute summer diarrhoea of infective origin affecting both child and adult alike. The most vulnerable patient is always the small infant because of the dangers of dehydration from severe vomiting or diarrhoea. When this is suspected the child must be hospitalised immediately, having been given Rescue Remedy 5 drops before the ambulance arrives. The main symptoms are vomiting and diarrhoea, with fever, collapse and exhaustion. The attack may follow eating ice cream or suspect food, and involve the entire family.

REMEDIES

Arsenicum, Sulphur, Podophyllum, China, Pulsatilla, Aconitum, Colcocynthum.

Formica Rufa (Red Ant)

Tincture of the crushed Red Ant. Valuable in rheumatic and gouty conditions with darting burning pains, headaches. Vagueness and lack of concentration. Facial Paralysis.

Fractures

These must of course be treated surgically in a specialised hospital unit. The remedy *Symphytum 6* supports natural repair once fixing and alignment has been established. Use *Arnica* for any shock or haemorrhage during orthopædic treatment.

Fraxinus Americanus (White Ash)

Tincture of the bark. Introduced by Compton Burnett. Indicated in uterine prolapse with bearing-down pains. *(Sepia).* Fibroids.

Frigidity

The common female condition of aversion to the sexual act with inability to achieve orgasm. The cause is always psychological, the roots deep and complex. Aversion to the sexual act may be quite unconscious, the cause traumatic in one form or other. The whole problem needs to be talked about and made less secret and less of an area of fear and failure. Where there is an on-going relationship with trust and sharing, without pressure to reach orgasm, then sexuality can be more relaxed.

Left to itself, it can recede into more overall patterns less of a life-and-death feature and criteria of success and acceptance. The whole mental and personality apsects of the woman has to be looked at with understanding, sometimes over a period of time. In all cases the 'power' of the symptom must be drawn by discussion and gentle exposure.

REMEDIES

Natrum Mur, Aconitum, Sepia, Silicea, Pulsatilla.

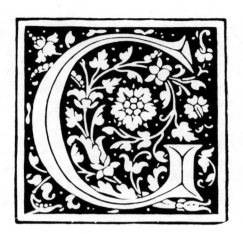

Gaertner (Morgan)

The bowel nosode, complimentary to Lycopodium. There is typically malnutrition and retarded stunted growth when indicated. Pale with blue eyes and freckles, usually highly intelligent but tense and nervous. Irritation of the renal tract is frequent with renal colic or recurrent cystitis. There are frequent gastro-intestinal problems of stomach ache, constipation, offensive diarrhoea, acidity, flatulence and vomiting. Threadworms.

Gait — awkward

For a variety of reasons the person is clumsy and awkward, lacking a movement which is upright and easy. One of the commonest causes is rheumatism or arthritis affecting the joints, and limiting movement. Other causes are hereditary disease, trauma, following any severe or chronic condition of the limbs or after a surgical intervention with shortening or fixation of a joint to lessen pain (arthrodesis). Psychological factors, especially hysterical in type are another common cause.

REMEDIES
Rhus Tox, Lycopodium, Phosphorus, Natrum Mur.

Ganglion

The common localised swelling of the wrist area due to thickening

of the tendon sheath causing pain or discomfort. The cause is unknown, but they seem to be related often to trauma.
REMEDIES
Ruta, Baryta Carb, Rhus Tox, Benz. Ac.

Gastritis

Inflammation of the lining mucosal layer of the stomach. The commonest cause is infective, but it may be associated with peptic ulceration, or irritation from a foreign body swallowed by a child. Major symptoms are pain and discomfort in the stomach region, the pain colicy in type with flatulence, sometimes nausea or vomiting.
REMEDIES
Nux Vom, Pulsatilla, Mag. Phos, Arsenicum, Sulphur, Belladonna.

Gelsemium (Yellow Jasmine)

Tincture of the root-bark. Introduced by Hale. Indicated for general infections of the influenzal type with marked lassitude, tremors and rigors. There is an irritable state of mind with aching generalised pains, collapse, weakness, trembling, diarrhoea and vomiting. Also of great value in hysteria, especially examination-fear and stage-fright. It is one of the most valuable and basic first-aid homoeopathic remedies.

Gentiana Cruciata (Cross-leaved Gentian)

Tincture of the root, first proved by Watzke. Indications include acute infections — especially of stomach and throat. Colic, vomiting with watery diarrhoea. Hernia.

Gentry, William. M.D. (–   )

The early American homeopath.
His major writings include:
(1875) *An answer to the question – What is Homoeopathy*
(1890) *The Concordance Repertory of the more characteristic symptoms of the Materia Medica*, in six volumes.
The rubrical and regional text-book of Homoeopathic Materia Medica.

Gingivitis

Inflammation of the gums, with softness, redness and sometimes bleeding.
REMEDIES
Hepar Sulph, Merc. Sol, Sulphur, Ac. Nit., Silicea.

Glaucoma

The acute or chronic condition of raised intra-ocular pressure, causing pain and visual disturbance. The condition is a serious one that requires specialist treatment, the cause often unknown.
REMEDIES
Ruta, Gelsemium, Natrum Mur.

Glonoin (Nitro-glycerine)

First proved by Hering. There are sudden violent pulsating heachaches with bursting throbbing pain, violent hot flushes, worse at night, drenching night sweats, fainting fits. All symptoms worse for the least jarring movement (*Belladonna*). A useful remedy for sunstroke.

Glossitis

Inflammation of the tongue, due to infection, trauma or from eating food which is too hot. The tongue is sore, red and may be swollen. Eating and swallowing are painful and uncomfortable.
REMEDIES
Rhus Tox (when the area affected is the tip),
Arnica (from trauma),
Apis (when there is swelling),
Ac. Nit., (when there is blistering of the sides of the tongue and mouth),
Natrum Mur (when follows a bee sting. (Also give *Apis.*)

Gnaphalium (Everlasting flower, cud-weed)

A remedy for sciatic nerve irritation — either left or right, worse at night. Lumbago. Numbness is an indication to prescribe which alternates with the pain. Colicy diarrhoea, throughout the day, irritability, dysmenorrhoea.

Goitre

Swelling of the thyroid may be the result of glandular over-activity-causing a toxic condition with loss of weight, tremor, protruberent eyeballs, with exhaustion, or it may be due to a simple goitre provoked by the lack of mineral Iodine in the diet. The toxic goitre is most serious needing urgent treatment. Danger from a goitre may be mechanical apart from the underlying thyroid disturbance, due to pressure on the oesophagus or windpipe causing difficulty with swallowing or shortness of breath where the swelling is located behind the sternum.

REMEDIES
Natrum Mur for toxic goitre.
Thyroideum for single goitre or thyroid deficiency, e.g. postoperatively.

Gout

Inflammation of the proximal or first great toe joint from unknown reasons. Uric acid crystals tend to deposit in the area affected and the blood level is raised. Symptoms are pain, swelling with redness and often considerable irritability. The cause is often over-rich living with excesses of meat and wine.

REMEDIES
Colchicum 6 hourly, *Aconite, Nux Vom, Belladonna.*

Graphites (Black pencil lead)

Trituration of black pencil lead. One of Hahnemann's most valuable and important anti-Psora remedies. Particularly valuable in skin problems especially acne, psoriasis and eczema. Erruptions and irritating lesions which exude a clear, straw-coloured fluid and are often typically behind the ears. It is particularly indicated for the obese, chilly type of make-up with frequent nose-bleeds, itching and weakness. The personality is over-sensitive, especially to music, weeping easily, depressed and exhausted by colicy pains, mucous diarrhoea and general loss of reserves and vigour.

Grauvogl, Von Edward, M.D. (1811-1877)

The 19th Century German homoeopath, who practised in

Nuremburg.
Major writings include:
1870 *Textbook of Homoeopathy*
1879 *The homoeopathic law of similarities.*

Grief (effects of)

Suppressed grief is one of the most undermining and damaging of all psychological conditions. It not only contributes to depression but may also provoke reactions of guilt, loss of confidence, fatigue and a variety of recurrent physical conditions that are resistance to all treatments. Such physical symptoms may recur yearly the time or date of the loss (anniversary reactions).
REMEDIES
Ignatia, Natrum Mur.

Grimmer, Arthur Hill. M.D. (1874–1967)

The American homoeopath, pupil and secretary to Kent, for many years, one of Kent's 'inner circle'. he was a graduate of the Chicago Hahnemann Medical College and a gifted homoeopath. He had known of the homoeopathic method since childhood and his parents' medical chest. He initially practised in Chicago, working closely with Kent on the Repertory. Later he lived in Florida and taught at the American Foundation of Homoeopathy for many years.

Guaiacum (Gum resin of the Lignum Vitae tree)

An anti-psora remedy acting especially on fibrous tissue, joints and ligaments. Also muscles and mucous membrane causing distortions and contractions in the area with deformity (compare *Causticum*). Useful in chronic gouty and rheumatic conditions with tearing shooting pains, contractions with stiffness and limitation of movement. Aggravated from movement, cold and damp.

Guernsey, Henry Newell. M.D. (1817–1885)

Born in Vermont and graduate from the New York University in 1842, Guernsey practised mainly in Philadelphia. Member of the American Institute of Homoeopathy in 1846, he was appointed professor of obstetrics at the Homoeopathic College of Pennsylvania in 1857. He was the first homoeopath to strongly and publicly advocate the single remedy and was significant in the introduction of high potencies.

His major writings include:

1865 *Introductory lectures on obstetrics and diseases of women and children*

1867 *Application of the homoeopathic principles and practise to obstetrics.*

1868 *The key-note system*

1870 *Uterine Haemorrhage*

1870 *The homoeopathic treatment of disordered dentition*

1870 *The homoeopathic materia medica*

1887 *Key-notes to the materia medica*

1877 *Ovarian tumours*

1882 *Plain talks on avoided subjects.*

Guernsey, William Jefferson. M.D. (1854–1935)

The American homoepathic physician and author.

Major writings include:

1879 *The Travellers medical repertory and family advisor for the homoeopathic tretment of acute disease.*

1882 *Haemorrhoids*

1883 *Desires and Aversions*

1885 *The Card Repertory*

1889 *Guernsey's Boenninghausen*

Gumboils

The recurrent infection of the gums with boil formation. The cause is often obscure, but frequently associated with a dental problem and infection at the dental-roots.

REMEDIES

Sulphur, Silicea, Merc. Sol, Phosphorus.

Gutman, William. M.D. (–   )

The eminent contemporary American homoeopath, active in New York, often as a solo voice for many years. A graduate of Vienna, Gutman has throughout his life been an enthusiastic supporter of research. President of the American Institute of

Homoeopathy 1965–66, chairman of the research council of the International League, he remains an active supporter of international provings and clinical research.

Haehl, Richard, M.D. (1873-1932)

The emminent German homoeopathic physician from Stutgart where he spent most of his working life. Member of the Homoeopathic Central society of Germany, honourary member of the Hahnemann College of Philadelphia and the North America Homoeopathic Society, he is most known for his excellent and comprehensive 2-volume biography of Hahnemann. From the year 1898, he collected all the letters, documents and papers he could, visiting relatives to compile a comprehensive background. He worked closely with Boenninghausen's wife and foster-daughter of Melanie — Hahnemann's second wife. He was also closely connected with the sixth edition of the *Organon,* writing the preface, helping to secure this most significant edition with its extensive footnotes.

Haemorrhoids (piles)

The common condition of piles due to varicosities of the anal venous supply, often associated with chronic contipation or following childbirth. Symptoms are mucous discharge, fresh blood on the stools and pain or irritation. Sometimes the pile may enlarge, becoming blue and painful to the extent of preventing sitting or comfort.

REMEDIES

Pulsatilla, Hamamelis, Aloes, Aesculus, Lachesis.

99

Hahnemann, Samuel (1755–1843)

The founder and father of homoeopathy. Born in Meissen, Germany, where his father and grandfather had worked as artist-painters to the porcelain industry. He was an outstanding scholar and scientist from an early age as well as a gifted linguist. His studies were varied in both Leipzig and Vienna which gave him a breadth of vision and a sensitivity which together with his knowledge and admiration for the philosophical works of Paracelsus led to his eventual insights and discoveries. The principles of homoeopathy occurred by chance when Hahnemann was translating the works of Cullen in 1790. He took some Cinchona bark — the active ingredient of Quinine and to his astonishment, being in good health, developed all the symptoms of an acute intermittent, malarial-type of febrile illness. From these chance beginnings, Hahnemann tested or 'proved over 100 new remedies with his proving group of dedicated doctors as well as himself and family. This led into the Law of Similars or the principle of *Simila Similibus Curentur* — 'Let like be treated by like' which is the cornerstone of the method. He advocated that the remedy be taken in the smallest or single dosage for cure, the remedies to be prepared quite uniquely by a combination of serial dilution and succussion at every stage. His theory of vital energy is amply described in his classic treatise the *Organon*. A contemporary of Goethe and anticipating Jung by 100 years, like Freud, Hahnemann knew the significance of the psychological as well as the importance of the seemingly paradoxal stimulant to cause a physiological response or reaction which both Goethe and Jung advocated at different periods and in different ways. Beset by opposition and criticism at many periods of his life, Hahnemann remained a tireless researcher, physician and teacher.

His major writings include:

1793 *Pharmaceutical dictionary, Materia Medica Pura*

1810 *Organon,* revised six times in as many editions

1828 *Chronic disease* in four volumes.

Appropriately and aptly on his Pierre Lachaise (Paris) tombstone are engraved in Latin — *Non Inutile Vixi* — I have not lived in vain.

Hair Problems

Commonly seen in the surgery for many reasons including hair-loss (see section *Alopoecia*), or because the hair is thin, lacks vitality, or is greasy. The hair is an extension of the outer layer of the skin and is a reflection of the basic health and vitality of the individual. Its vitality, lustre, bounce and general health may be affected by any upset to the system — including nutritional, hormonal, psychological or infective. The health of the hair is inseparable from the health of the scalp and when this is affected, the hair is also less healthy.

REMEDIES

Bryonia, for dry hair often patchy,

Silicea, when the hair is weak or brittle, splitting and lacking vigour,

Arsenicum for premature greyness,

Lycopodium for premature hair loss.

China for weakness of growth after a prolonged and weakening illness,

Sulphur when associated with an infected scalp.

Natrum Mur or *Lycopodium* hair loss due to tnesion and anxiety.

Hale, Edwin M. (1829–1899)

The American 19th century homoeopath who introduced a whole series of new and valuable remedies to homoeopathy. These include *Gelsemium, Hydrastis, Iberis, Lycopus, Passiflora, Phytolacca, Plantago*. Hale was professor of the Hahnemann's college of Chicago.

Major writings include:

Materia Medica

(1875) *Specific Therapeutics of the New Remedies*

Hammamelis (Witch Hazel)

A circulatory remedy with special action on venous flow. Proved by Hering. Extremely valuable in varicose conditions, haemorrhoids and phlebitis or conditions where there is stasis and congestion with pain and swelling. Indicated for haemorrhages from piles, menopausal flooding, also post-operatively.

101

Harmony

That aspect of man which is the basis of all relaxation and true health. It is the essence of internal vital balance which homoeopathy aims to restore and maintain and includes harmony at both mental as well as physical levels. Its presence is largely dependent on an uninterrupted flow of vital energy and when this is blocked or not available — usually from stress causes, then disharmony occurs and the struggles of the organism to correct and balance itself is often manifested externally as symptoms.

Hartmann, Franz. M.D. (1796–1853)

The early German Homoeopath, born in Delitsch. One of Hahnemann's 'provers union', the original group of physicians, including Stapf, who worked in the development of new remedies and the repertory. He worked mainly in Leipsic and remained one of Hahnemann's earliest disciples and friend.
Writings include:
1841 *Practical observations of some chief homoeopathic remedies*
1847 *Hartmann's theory of acute disease and homoeopathic treatment*
1849 *Hartmann's theory of chronic disease and homoeopathic treatment*
1853 *Diseases of children and their homoeopathic treatment.*

Hawkes, Alfred Edward. M.D. (1849–1919)

The Edinburgh graduate and homoeopathic physician, mainly of women's diseases. He worked most of his life in Liverpool where he was physician to the Hahnemann Hospital. Introduced to homoeopathy by Dr. Arthur Clifton of Northampton, he was a tireless worker and active to the journals and societies.
Major writings include:
1913 *Mucous colitis treated with iso-tonic sea-water*
1914 *Notes on a case treated with Tuberculinum*
1814 *Gastric Ulcers*
1916 *Retroversion of the gravid uterus.*
Other papers were written on the Heart, Addison's disease, Alcohol, Seborrhoea.

Headaches

The common condition of head pains, either periodic and starting on one side as with migraine, or a more generalised pain, which is vague and varies in position from one attack to the next. When they are recurrent, it is important to find the underlying cause which can vary from overwork, poor light condition, inadequate air and ventilation to dietary excess or infection. Visual causes, where a change of glasses is needed, require a check-up by an optician. There are many psychological reasons for headaches. The attacks may also have commenced after a trauma or accident, often provoked by a problem in the cervical vertebrae, which needs correction. Another common cause is catarrh and recurrent sinusitis. In all cases a proper diagnosis and full investigation is required as part of the homoeopathic approach to rule-out underlying pathology that requires surgical or an alternative approach to the homeopathic one — the patients needs come first — before than any desire by the physician to prescribe. Having made the diagnosis we can then consider the best treatment for the individual patient and his particular headache.

REMEDIES

Silicea when the pain begins in the occipital region and radiates forwards over the skull.

Lycopodium when the pain is mainly situated in the right temple region, worse in the afternoon between 4–8.00.

Kali Carb when the pain is more often left-sided, in the mornings or late evenings, drawing in type, and aggravated by airless conditions.

Pulsatilla where the pain is variable, worse for heat, without thirst.

Aconite for very acute painful attacks.

Nux Vom when there is irritability and the headache follows a period of dietary indiscretion.

Coffea, when there is severe pain, restlessness, and there has been considerable abuse of coffee over the years.

Health

That subtle and harmonious condition which is the aim of the homoeopathic physician with freedom from dis-ease. Well-being and relaxation at both physical and psychological levels within the person.

Heat

Always to be avoided in excess, especially when the person is in a fatigued or convalescent state. Where there is particular intolerance of heat in any form consider *Pulsatilla, Arg. Nit.* or *Sulphur* as possible remedies. Craving for heat — the person cold on the warmest day, consider *Arsenicum* or *Calcarea* as possible remedies.

Helleborus Niger (Christmas Rose)

Tincture of the fresh root — the 'niger' — referring to its black colour. There is considerable irritability with shooting headaches and inability to concentrate. Indicated for old or recent head injuries where headaches, personality changes, epilepsy with convulsions have occurred. The headache and giddyness is aggravated by movement and the least draught of cool air.

Hempel, Charles Julius (1811–1879)

The emminent homoeopathic writer and physician of Prussian origin. He studied and travelled widely in Paris and elsewhere before finally settling in the U.S. in 1835 where he studied medicine. Co-editor of the *Homoeopathic Examiner* 1843–45, professor of materia medica and therapeutics at the Philadelphia medical college, translator of some of Hahnemann's most important works into English.

His writings include:

1845 *A treatise on the use of Arnica in contusions, wounds and sprains*
1846 *The Homoeopathic domestic physician*
1853 *A complete repertory of the homoeopathic materia medica*
1854 *Organon of specific homoeopathy*
1859 *A new and comprehensive system of materia medica and therapeutics*
1860 *Homoeopathy, a principle of nature*
1867 *Lectures on homoeopathy*
1868 *The new remedies*
1874 *The science of homoeopathy*
1880 *Materia medica and therapeutics*

Henderson, William. M.D. (1811–1872)

The Edinburgh graduate and later Professor of pathology at the university of Edinburgh who gained prominence by developing a rational and scientific status for homoeopathy by his brilliant attention to research and detail. He was disapproved of by many contemporaries because they considered he was trying to make homoeopathy popular by emphasising physical signs and pathology, rather than an overall symptom-profile of the patient. He tried to develop remedies for certain illness-conditions like bronchitis and pneumonia and was supported in this pathological approach by Hughes.

His writings include:

Homoeopathy fairly represented — in reply to Dr. Simpson's *Homoeopathy – misrepresented.*
1845 *Homoeopathic practise.*

Hepar Sulph (Sulphide of Calcium)

Prepared by burning the middle layer of the oyster shell with flowers of sulphur. It is an ancient remedy, proved by Hahnemann and indicated for chronic gouty conditions. There is over-sensitivity to both touch and cold air with marked irritability and exhaustion. It is an excellent remedy for infection, especially of the upper respiratory tract, tonsils, larynx and bowels. Indicated for offensive purulent conditions and painful infections with foul-smelling discharges, diarrhoea, urinary infections.

Hepatitis

The acute viral infection. Frequently contageous, passed by sexual contact, or carriers who transmit the viral infection but are themselves apparently symptom-free.

REMEDIES
Phosphorus, Chelidon, Sulphur, Croton Tig, Bryonia, Hepar Sulph.

Hering, Dr. Constantine (1800–1880)

The emminent pioneer of homoeopathy in the U.S.A. He began his career as an opponent of homoeopathy, but on trying the remedies and theories in practise, he became its most active and

105

ardent supporter both in Dresden and Philadelphia. He founded the Hahnemann Medical College in 1836. Instrumental in proving and introducing *Lachesis,* the Bushmaster or Surucucu snake remedy into homoeopathy. His great literary achievement was *Guiding Symptoms* in 10 volumes.

Hering's Law

During the course of homoeopathic treatment, symptoms improve from above downwards; from the most vital to less vital organs; from most recent to earliest symptoms and in reverse order of appearance.

Hernia

In general this is best treated surgically rather than by a truss or support because of the danger of strangulation or cutting-off the blood supply to the intestine within the hernia. Surgery may not always be possible for reasons of general health or unavailable when homoeopathy is indicated.

REMEDIES
Nux. Vomica, Calcarea, Lycopodium.

Herpes Zoster (Shingles)

The common infection of the elderly with a chicken-pox type of virus. Second attacks can occur though not very commonly. Any nerve-root may be involved in the infection — usually of the abdominal region but at times the spinal nerve roots of the skull or the orbit are invaded affecting vision. There is severe pain, irritation, itching, blistering and typical scarring. Healing may take several months for full recovery with neuralgic pain. Homoeopathy is very effective.

REMEDIES
Rhus Tox, Ranunculus Bulb, Natrum Mur.

Hiatus Hernia

The common condition of herniation of part of the stomach into the chest cavity alongside the oesophagus because of weakness — usually congenital, of the diaphragm muscle. The condition is not serious but it can be the cause of much discomfort, pain and heart-burn, particularly on bending or when there has been a

106

change of posture. If severe, surgical repair of the weak area of the diaphragm may be required.

REMEDIES

Nux Vom. is often very helpful.

Hip Problems

These are usually either arthritic or traumatic or more rarely infective in origin.

REMEDIES

Rhus Tox when the condition is aggravated by cold and damp and better for movement.

Ruta often improved by humidity and one of the best large-joint remedies.

Mercurius for infective conditions as osteomyelitis.

Hippocrates (460–377 B.C.)

The famous Greek physician, born at Cos, father of modern medicine, who introduced the famous Hippocratic Oath for all practising doctors. Hippocrates was first to notice the homoeopathic principle that like cures like over 2,000 years ago.

Homoeopathy

The system of medicine that treats the patient as an individual in its approach to the totality of the person, not just treating symptoms in isolation as if they were external, foreign things, unrelated to the psychology, constitutional and vital make-up of the person. Symptoms themselves are regarded as a key part of health rather than of disease and seen as the healthy response to underlying dis-ease and an essential part of cure. This vital symptom-response is supported by the homoeopathic remedies which are given in minute quantities in order to encourage and stimulate the body's intrinsic and natural vital response. Most of the remedies are of plant, mineral or animal origin and have been 'proved' on healthy human volunteers to give a profile of symptoms which can be matched by the homoeopath to those of the individual patient. The correct remedy is one which in its natural and usually toxic form would stimulate a reaction similar to one which is the object of treatment. Suppression and blockage of symptoms by any method is regarded as dangerous to the patient, pushing the true problem 'underground' and not really curing the underlying cause because the emphasis is on the complaint only and not the underlying reasons for it. Usually the homoeopathic remedy is given in a single dose or when repeated, it is stopped as soon as there is marked improvement in the patient's well-being and symptom-response. Homoeopathy was founded by Hahnemann at the end of the 18th century in the face of enormous opposition from conventional medicine who accused it of being 'unscientific'. Such opposition has continued until fairly recent years. Now it is much more accepted by the establishment and has finally begun to gain recognition in universities and medical schools of Europe as a 'respectable' speciality. But the fight for recognition has been long and there are still echoes of it in a few quarters. Each year more and more medical men are being thoroughly trained in homoeopathy, but the numbers of doctors is still insufficient as the demand increases by thinking patients who want a viable safe alternative method of prevention and cure.

Hubbard-Wright, Elizabeth M.D. (1896–1967)

The New York born graduate of Columbia — one of the first women graduates, who specialised in homoeopathy in New York for most of her life. She was known as editor of *The Journal of the American Institute of Homoeopathy* and president of the institute from 1959/60. Author of *A Brief Study Course in Homoeopathy*.

Hughes, Richard. M.D. (1836–1902)

The emminent scholar and homoeopathic physician, working at the London Homoeopathic Hospital, although mainly based in Brighton with Madden, where he was physician to the Brighton Homoeopathic Dispensary. Hughes met with many critics, particularly because he was a 'low' potency prescriber and his insistance on prescribing by taking into account the site of action of the disease; the organs affected; the causative factors and the evolution of symptoms during an illness. He had a brilliant mind and his healthy questioning of dogmatic attitudes earned him many enemies. His fault was that he tried to popularise homoeopathy by making it more allopathic, emphasising the physical and pathological, rather overall than individual symptoms, the modalities and the individualisation of the method. By trying to make homoeopathy more 'scientific' and respectable he was in danger of undermining the whole approach. Henderson, Dudgeon and Hughes were all advocates of low potency prescribing only. All of this caused an enormous rift in the profession, particularly from his former friend Clarke and they became bitter opponents; Clarke accused him of pandering to the allopaths. In a recent (1980) Richard Hughes lecture, Anthony Campbell called for a fairer appraisal and review of Hughes contributions.

His major writings include:

1881 *Hahnemann as a medical philosopher*
   Knowledge of the physician
   Manual of Pharmaco-Dynamics
   Manual of therapeutics
   Principle and practise of homoeopathy, in 4 volumes — his major contribution
1886 *Cyclopædia of Drug Pathogenesy and repertory*

Hydrastis Canadensis (Golden seal)

Tincture of the fresh root. Proved by Hale. Indicated in chronic catarrhal conditions where there is a thick yellow tenacious sticky and stringy muduced. Reputedly of value as a prophylactic in pre-cancerous conditions. When there is general ill-health and vague symptoms of malaise.

Hyoscyamus Niger (Henbane)

Tincture of the fresh plant. One of the major mental remedies for mental excitement with overactivity, delirium, delusional behaviour. The face is pale often twitching with emotion and irritability. There is intolerance to any form of covering although the patient is chilly. It is often used with *Belladonna* in treatments but has less violence and redness.

Hypericum Perforatum (St. John's Wort)

Tincture of the whole fresh plant, first proved by Müllen. One of the major first-aid remedies for lacerating wounds with lancing, tearing, stabbing pains shooting up the limb and sensitive to the least touch. Indicated where there is damage to nerve tissue, either bruised or severed, particularly of skin, nails, hands or feet.

Hysterical Problems

In this much-maligned disease, there is displacement of psychological energy into the physical with the appearance of 'conversion' symptoms, which may be odd and bizarre — or more often resistant to all attempts to cure. The patient may be of any age, of either sex. Beneath the surface there are problems of security and often of sexuality, which is seen only in infantile terms. Frequently there is an old problem of ambivalent attachment to one of the parents — never resolved since childhood. The hysterical disturbance tends unfortunately to effect every aspect of living and relationships, with problems of fridigity, impotence, avoidance of the opposite sex or by contrast, provocation, and a tendency to be on display at all times. This helps compensate for feelings of inadequacy, yet at the same time making the most ordinary everyday happening an 'event' and a cause for tension.

REMEDIES

Pulsatilla, Natrum Mur, Ignatia, Gelsemium, Arg. Nit.

Iberis (Bitter Candytuft)

Tincture of the seed, introduced by Hale, as one of his new remedies. Primarily a cardiac remedy, it is of special value in angina where there is pain on effort, palpitations and distress. Vertigo with nausea, asthma, Meniere's Disease are other indications.

Ignatia (St. Ignatius Bean)

Tincture of the bean. Indicated for suppressed grief and loss-reactions, the patient never well since a bereavement or shock. Anal cramps and spasms with haemorrhoids are common. The mental state is one of tearfulness, anxiety and often globus hystericus (sensation of a lump in the throat).

Immunity to Drugs

Immunity to modern drugs can now be developed so rapidly by the most recent strains of bacteria and viral organisms that it takes them less time to become resistant than for the pharmaceutical industry to develop yet another more powerful antibiotic to try and destroy them. Hence the folly of developing more and more powerful drugs with massive prescribing — using a sledge hammer to kill an ant, with ever present dangers of totally resistant new strains emerging — the super virus or bacteria. Diseases like Legionnaires Disease, with no known treatment is

113

but one example of such wrong thinking with the emergence of seemingly incurable diseases, hitherto unknown. In many hospital wards, the presence of highly virulent strans makes them some of the least healthy and most dangerous places in Britain — as many patients know to their cost, with sudden severe infections occurring in an environment that should be the most safe and healthy. Some wards have to be completely closed down every years for several weeks or months for just this reason.

In homoeopathy such problems do not arise. There is not the obsession with developing more and more powerful remedies to the patient's cost in health. There is no danger of provoking new and more dangerous strains of organism in our environment, with emphasis on improving the 'soil' or individual resistance and innate resilience of the patient to stress — whatever its type. Conservation of reserves and vital energy must be maintained at all costs for health to be regained or preserved.

Impatience

One of the most severe and damaging problems of our present generation and society. Remedies 'in a hurry' where time seems to pass too slowly include *Medorrhinum, Aurum Met., Lil. Tig., Natrum Mur., Nux Vom.* The opposite where time passes too quickly and there is never enough time for anything indicates *Cococulus.*

Impetigo

The severe skin infection with pus formation, infection, swelling and redness, pain, temperature and discomfort. It can occur typically in debilitated adults or children. Although less common than previously it can still at times reach epidemic proportions and be highly infective.

REMEDIES
Merc. Sol., Sulphur, Arsenicum.

Impotence

The common male sexual problem. The causes are complex and often obscure, including hormonal, nutritional, toxic iatrogenic (drug side-effect), degenerative in the elderly. But most of all the psychological plays a role to some degree in every case because of the highly emotional nature and associations of the problem. Like its opposite-number and female-equivalent — frigidity, the underlying psychological factors, when present must come to the surface, be explored and discussed with distortions and apprehensions sympathetically understood. A true hormonal deficiency needs replacement therapy in addition to the homoeopathic approach.

REMEDIES

Lycopodium, Agnus Cast, Selenium, Natrum Mur.

Inbalance

Inbalance of the human organism at deepest level, manifesting as malaise, fatigue, and illness on the surface is what the homoeopathic prescription aims to correct. When there is inbalance from whatever cause, vital energy fails to function and flow freely and totally is blocked or displaced contributing to many patient-symptoms. With the correct homoeopathic remedy in potency, such inbalance and blockage can be slowly adjusted.

Incontinence

Lack of control of urinary flow often with loss of sphincter tone. The problem is a complex one. The cause may be traumatic after childbirth, or associated with uterine mal-position or prolapse. Infection, or degenerative changes in the elderly male or female also provkes weakness of the sphincter muscles.

REMEDIES

Causticum, Sepia, Sabal Serr., Baryta Carb.

Indications for the Remedy

These are the totality of symptoms of the patient, the modalities or aggravating and ameliorating features, any precipitating causes or anticedants such as vaccination — where the patient has never been well since that time.

Indigestion

One of the major illness-problems of our present society. The symptoms are pain, heartburn, acidity, and flatulence. For the majority there is underlying stress. Meals taken are usually of poor quality, eaten too quickly without adequate time or enjoyment so that proper secretion of digestive juices fails to occur and excessive acidity plays havoc with stomach and duodenal lining. Acute infection with nausea or diarrhoea may also complicate matters.

REMEDIES

Nux. Vom., Ornithogalum, Lycopodium, Arsenicum, Carbo Veg, Natrum Mur.

Individual — the patient as an

In Homoeopathy the patient is not a disease entity to be 'neutralised' or hammered by massive doses of modern drugs at all costs. Hahnemann considered that the patient was first of all a spirit, then a mind and only lastly a body and that treatment must be directed at all three elements in order for cure to be complete. Only the homoeopathic remedy is uniquely active in all three layers.

Individualisation of the Homoeopathic Approach

One of the most characteristic features of homoeopathy is that the patient is not just treated as a collection of problems and sickness symptoms. Each person is unique and different and expresses an underlying malaise or infection — even in an epidemic, in their unique individual way. Each requires a different remedy from the other as they present and experience their illness differently with varying areas of emphasis, anxiety and severity. Even identical twins with a seeming identical cold or sore throat, often have quite contrasting symptoms which indicate different prescriptions. This individualisation rather than a 'nuts and bolts', in for service' approach characterises the homoeopathic emphasis from the first consultation onwards. It is the individual that matters, (not even homoeopathy) — how best to help the person, even where an entirely different approach may be indicated. Homoeopathy is about people first, their individual needs, feelings and ideals, even more than it is about homoeopathic principles and remedies.

116

Infinitesimal dosage of Homoeopathy

This is not the basis of homoeopathy although many quite wrongly see is as synonymous with the method. It was developed late in the history of homoeopathy, mainly in America and many years after Hahnemann and it is not essential to the homoeopathic principle — more funamentally based on the Law of Similitudes and prescribing the simillimum remedy on the basis of the patient's total symptoms. Even if the remedy were not diluted at all, provided that it is prescribed on the basis of treating 'like by like', it would still be homoeopathic. Hahnemann for many years used mother tinctures of the remedies, but obtained side-effects which concerned him. It was only then that he began to experiment with diluting the remedies. He found by chance that instead of reducing the action and effectiveness of the remedy, it was further increased — not only safer for the patient, but wider and deeper in action. This troubled Hahnemann for many years as he could not understand how a process of dilution could apparently be continued to infinity, provided it was succussed or vitalised and still give more power to the remedy. He himself stopped at the 30c potency for most of his remedies and it was left to the American school to develop the 200c and M potencies at a much later stage. For further general comments see section Scientific. It is important to be quite clear that all the potencies and infinitesimal dosages, higher than the 12C do not contain any material presence of mother substance in the diluant. Such dilutions, although unique to homoeopathy, are not the fundamental principle of the method and even Hahnemann had his doubts as to their validity and efficiency — especially of the very high potencies. In recent years their clinical value has however been proved by their enormous value in chronic problems, resistant to all other means also in constitutional prescribing.

Influenza   See section 'Flu

Influenzinum (The Nosode of 'Spanish' Influenza)

The extract of the 1918/19 epidemic. Use the 30th potency and repeat hourly in severe cases. Can also be used for the common cold or coryza when the 30c potency should be taken three times a week. Symptoms are weakness, collapse, muscle and joint pains, sore throat, catarrh and cough. In an epidemic it can be given prophylactically either to give full protection or a modified course of illness.

Insect Remedies

The major insect remedies are *Apis* (Bee), *Cantharis* (Spanish Fly), *Formica Rufa* (the Red Ant).

Insomnia

The common problem of lack of sleep from impaired natural sleep rhythm often caused by abuse of sedative drugs over a period which has eroded the natural rhythms. We all need sleep for rest and to survive and underlying causes mut be clearly ascertained and corrected. The excessive use of addictive, dependency drugs must be removed so that sleep can again take on a natural pattern.

REMEDIES

Lycopodium when there is difficulty in getting off because of an over-active mind and fear of the future.

Aconite where insomnia is due to or provoked by fear.

Arsenicum when the person wakes just after midnight or in the early hours about 1.00 a.m.

Pulsatilla when insomnia is due to getting over-heated in bed and then feeling chilly, never really comfortable at any time or for that matter in any situation.

Kali Carb. when the person wakes between 3.00 and 5.00 a.m., falling asleep exhausted just before the alarm rings.

Nux. Vom. From dietary causes and late ill-balanced meals.

Coffea Caused by abuse of tea or coffee over a prolonged period.

International League of Homoeopathy

The co-ordinating body, formed in 1925, which sets the international standards for homoeopathy throughout the world and organises the international congresses, acting as a liasing body for the whole of the profession. Representatives of each country meet regularly to maintain high standards and co-ordination of research.

The president members of the council (1983) are:
Dr. R. Fleury (treasurer), Dr. W. Gutman (Nat. Vice president),
Dr. F. Lamasson (president), Dr. S. Ortega (Nat. Vice president),
Dr. T. Paschero (Nat. Vice president), Dr. L. P. Schmidt
(president of Honour).

Iodium (the element of Iodine)

Iodine in tincture. Works best for dark-complexioned people
where there is wasting and thinness of limbs. Chronic infections,
stroke or arthritis. Restless and excitable. Useful in pneumonia
with shortness of breath and cough. Fatigue, weakness and
faintness are other common features and indications.

Ipecacuanha (the Ipecac plant)

Tincture of the whole root. Nausea with vomiting, salivation,
disgust for food, depression are the major indications.
Congestion is rampant with a loud rattling loose cough, the chest
moist, congested with breathing difficult. The patient is often
sitting-up, sometimes fighting for breath. Whooping cough,
breathless from excess of fluid and mucous in the chest, cardiac
failure, haemorrhage, threatened abortion, are the other
indications.

Iris Versicolor (the Blue Flag)

Tincture of the fresh root. First introduced by Kitchen. An early
North American Indian remedy. It acts primarily on the
alimentary tract. Severe burning pains, particularly of mouth and
stomach, vomiting, watery diarrhoea, colic, right-sided migraine
are the major indications to prescribe.

Iritis

Inflammation of the ocular Iris. For any acute inflammatory
infections of the eye which do not resolve rapidly always consult a
specialist-practitioner in order to avoid the dangers of chronic
problems developing and the risk of permanent damage to vision.
REMEDIES
Merc. Sol., Rhus Tox, Sulphur, Duboisia.

Irritability

The common temperamental problem. In some cases provoked by trauma or concussion with a change of personality, or in others an expression of underlying depression and feelings of inadequacy.

The major remedies are *Nux. Vom., Chamomilla, Staphisagria, Cina, Colocynth, Hepar Sulph.*

'Itch' The

The 'Itch' or Psora, now most commonly seen as Psoriasis is the common miasm described by Hanemann as the major underlying hereditary cause of chronic disease in our modern society. See *'Psora'* section for greater detail.

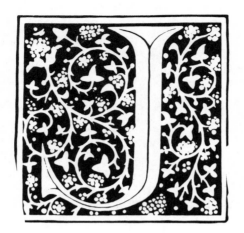

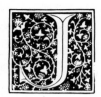

Jaundice

Abnormal accumulation of bile salts particularly bilirubin in the blood stream, causing the characteristic yellow discolouration. The cause is either blockage of the bile duct which normally discharges into the intestine and gives the characteristic colour to the stool, as from gall stones or the problem may be in the liver itself, due to cell-blockage as from infective hepatitis, or certain tropical diseases. In the young baby the cause may be a high level of blood cells which are abnormally fragile from sensitivity to an inherited Rhesus factor from one parent. Infantile jaundice is dealt with by exchange transfusion when necessary. If mild it resolves spontaneously within a few days. Accurate diagnosis is essential.

REMEDIES

Phosphorus, China, Chelidonium, Sulphur, Cholesterinum.

Jahr, George Heinrich Gottleib. M.D. (1800–1875)

Born in Saxony, Jahr had a most emminent and successful medical career as a homoeopath, particularly associated with the spread and development of homoeopathic principles in Europe, perhaps secondary only in importance to Hahnemann himself. He qualified in Bonn, but worked for most of his life in France and the bulk of his extensive practise and writing was done in Paris. His output was prolific, sound and thoughtful. Major written contributions are:

1836 *Manual of Homoeopathic medicine* (4 volumes)
1841 *Jahr's new manual of homoeopathic practise*
1839 *Elementary notions of homoeopathy*
1845 *Jahr's symptom codex* (or digest of symptoms)
1850 *A new homoeopathic pharmacopoeia*
1850 *Alphabetical repertory of skin symptoms*
1850 *Jahr's clinical guide and pocket repertory*
1856 *Nervous derangements and mental disease*
1856 *The homoeopathic treatment of female disease*
1868 *The venereal diseases*
1869 *Forty years of practise.*

Jealousy

The common emotional state based on insecurity and loss of confidence. There is obsessional fear of loss associated with possessiveness. The preoccupation is always the same — another person is a threat because of their beauty, wealth, sexuality, position, success, youth, intelligence, or any attribute that they seem to have more of. At the same time, there is under-valuing of the self, impairing confidence, relaxation and a mature acceptance of life's inevitable differences — the gains and losses, movement and change and seeming inequality — often felt to be unjust. Exploration of underlying fears, lack of confidence and any early traumas should be combined with the homoeopathic remedy. The following recommended remedies all have features which are relevant to the problem. *Apis, Lachesis, Staphisagria, Hyoscyamus, Natrum Mur, Pulsatilla.*

Jenichen, Julius, M.D. (1787-1845)

The early practitioner and researcher who first developed the M.M. potency.

Julien, Frederick Bennet. M.D. (–   )

The homoeopathic physician, trained at Cork who spent much of his active professional life on the staff of the Liverpool Hahnemann Hospital and dispensary since 1921. He died at the age of 65.

124

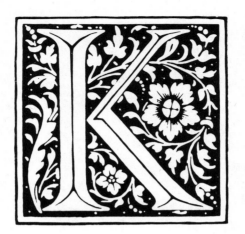

Kafka, Jakob D., M.D. (1809-1893)

The emminent early19th century German homoeopath and editor of the *Allgmeine Hom. Zeitung* 1872.

Kali Bic (Bicarbonate of Potassium)

First proved by Drysdale in 1844. One of the major polycrest remedies of value in conditions with stringy, yellow, mucoid-purulent discharges particularly of nose and throat or where localised 'small spot' pains occur. Ulceration of skin, bone or mucous membrane is an indication for the remedy, as too a sore throat, with the sensation of a 'hair on the back of the tongue'. It is particularly indicated for obese, fair-haired people, lacking in energy and vitality.

Kali Brom. (Potassium Bromide)

Restless depression with exhaustion, impotency, chronic acne and nenopausal flooding are the major indications.

Kali Carb (Potassium Carbonate)

The polycrest remedy for restless anxiety, depression and fear of solitude. Basically a left-sided remedy it acts strongly on mucous membrane of throat and alimentary tract with chronic catarrh, indigestion wth heartburn, and stich-like rheumatic pains.

Asthma and hay-fever. All symptoms worse from 3–5.00 a.m. is characteristic.

Kali Iod. (Potassium Iodide)

Loss of weight with palpitations, nodular skin eruptions, ulcerative and offensive purulent discharges. Depression with anxiety is common also chest infections particularly bronchitis, pneumonia and asthma.

Kali Phos. (Potassium Phosphate)

Introduced by Schuessler into Homoeopathy and proved .by Allen. There is nervous restless depression with weakness or paralysis and yellowish discharges. Tremor with numbness is a feature and it is particularly indicated after shock or convalescence. Amenorrhoea, laryngitis, insomnia, with craving for ice-cold drinks and foods are other prescribing features.

Kali Sulph. (Potassium Sulphate)

Introduced by Schuessler and indicated for infected skin conditions with yellowish discharges as erysipilas. Chronic nasal and bronchial conditions with catarrhal discharges. Measles, scarlet fever. Rheumatism. Better for fresh air and aggravated by heat is characteristic of all symptoms.

Kalmia Latifolia (N. American Laurel)

Tincture of the fresh leaves in flower and proved by Hering. A valuable right-sided remedy particularly for problems of severe facial pain and neuralgia. Angina, palpitations, shingles, wandering rheumatic pains, spinal paralysis with weakness of legs and lack of balance. Worse for cold, movement or touch, are characteristic indications to prescribe.

Kent, James Tyler. M.D. (1849–1916)

Born in Woodhull, New York, Kent was certainly one of the most emminent of all American homoeopaths. He practised mainly in Philadelphia and St. Louis. An able teacher, he was professor of materia medica at the homoeopathic college of St. Louis from

1881–88. Professor of materia medica and dean of the post-graduate school of homoeopathy, Philadelphia 1889–90. Professor of materia medica, Hering medical school, Chicago 1903–1910. Member of the American Institute of Homoeopathy, the International Hahnemann Association and founder of the society of Homoeopathians. Kent particularly advocated the single remedy and to wait before all improvement had ceased before repeating the dosage or remedy. He was instrumental in encouraging high potency prescribing and he proved many new remedies. He was a great teacher, and some of our greatest prescribers have studied under him, including Weir, Borland, Clarke, Schmidt. He did more than anyone to bring homoeopathy back from being popularised and lessened by polypharmacy and prescriptions based on pathology alone. He advocated strict Hahnemann studies. For chronic problems, he adovcated the 200c potency or above to resolve it.

His major writings include:

1877 *Repertory of homoeopathic materia medica – his greatest contribution*

1900 *Homoeopathic Philosophy – a fundamental statement of homoeopathic principles.*

1905 *Lectures on homoeopathic materia medica* — this book is still widely used by students and practitioners and has become a classic reference volume.

Keratosis

The common condition of the skin due either to aging or excessive exposure to the sun over prolonged periods. There are small isolated greyish elevated areas irregular in shape and unsightly on either the backs of the hands or face. They are of cosmetic importance only rather than of medical significance or a cause of discomfort.

REMEDIES

Sulphur, Ant. Crud., Nitric Ac.

Knee Problems

These are common at any age and in all cases a careful diagnosis must be made. Such problems are often arthritic or rheumatic in origin, but other causes as trauma, infection, sprain or degeneration must be excluded in every case. It is common to see the knee swollen in a severe rheumatic problems either involving the knee alone. or as part of a generalised joint inflammatory process. In the more simple and straightforward arthritic 'wear and tear' problems there is less inflammation and heat locally although the swelling may be just as severe. Pain is common and can come from joints or the ligaments with tear or strains being common. There may have been a fall with perhaps a fracture of the patella or tip of one of the long bones in the area. When in doubt an x-ray is always essential.

REMEDIES

Pulsatilla, Rhus Tox, Ruta, Sulphur, Apis, Symphytum.

Knerr, Calvin. B.M.D. (1847–1940)

The 19th Century American homoeopath.
His writings include:
1878 *Coup de Soleil'* or sunstroke with homoeopathic treatment.
He worked as co-editor of Hering's *Guiding Symptoms*.

Koch, Richard. M.D. (1849–1910)

The emminent American 19th century homeopath.
Writings include:
1867 *General address to the first Philadelphia Homoepathic medical college*
1871 *Valedictory address given to the Hahnemann Medical college.*

Korsakow dilution

One of the earliest methods of serial dilution to produce the homoeopathic potency. It has been much more popular on the continent than in the U.K. The principle is to prepare the potencies by using the same recipient for each subsequent dilution rather than a set of different glass tubes. The Korsakow method assumes that in the centisimal dilution, when the container is emptied, one drop of dilution remains adhered to the surface of the container so that the addition of 99 drops each time gives the correct C potency. Although widely used at one time, it is now out of favour and generally considered to be inferior to using individual separate phials at each stage of dilution.

Kreosotum (Creosote or rectified spirits)

A valuable left-sided remedy for chronic infective conditions with purulent discharge, weakness and loss of weight. It is indicated for chronic gum problems, tooth decay, irritation of bladder or prostate from infective causes. Chronic skin infections with irritation and pus. Uterine infections with offensive discharges. Foul breath and tongue, vomiting, colic and an excessive canine appetite is typical of many psoric conditions and suggests the remedy.

Labyrinthitis

Acute infection or irritation of the inner ear, with severe giddyness, nausea, vomiting and exhaustion.

REMEDIES

Aconite (for acute attacks), *Cocculus, Sal. Ac. Cyclamen, Conium, Glonoin, Arg. Nit.*

Lac Caninum (Bitch's Milk)

One of the most ancient medical remedies, introduced to Homoeopathy by Reisig. It is of special value in diphtheria and severe sore throat. The pains alternate from one side to the other, with a bloody, purulent discharge, restlessness, anxiety and prostration. Typically there are fearful dreams and phobia of snakes.

Lacerations

These should be cleaned with calendula lotion and any bleeding stopped by pressure, with all foreign material cleaned out and thoroughly removed. If severe, suture of the area is needed.

REMEDIES

Hypericum for nerve damage or bruising with shooting pains.
Arnica for bruising and shock.
Ledum for small and clean penetrating wounds.
Ruta or *Bellis Perennis* for sprains.

135

Apis for bruising.
Phosphorus for bleeding or haemorrhage.

Lachesis (the Surukuku or Bushmaster Snake)

Introduced to homoeopathy and proved by Hering in one of the most dramatic and courageous of all proving.

Typically all symptoms are worse from sleep, with intolerance of tight-clothing in any form and very sensitive to touch. It is a left-sided remedy having many uterine symptoms, particularly severe haemorrhage and flooding, with bladder or rectal infection common.

Lachnantes (Red root)

A remedy for upper respiratory tract infections with dry sore throat, hoarseness, dry cough, rheumatism of the neck region with a stiff neck, rheumatism. (Compare *Causticum*).

Lamasson, F. R. D., M.D. (1907-1975)

The emminent French homoeopathic physician and teacher, formerly a pupil of Pierre Schmidt of Geneva. President currently of the International League; President of the French Society of Homoeopathy; President of the National Institute of French Homoeopathy.

Lapis Alb (Calcium Silico-Fluoride)

Introduced to homeopathy by Grauvogl. There are burning pains in the stomach, uterus and breasts. Of value in itchy skin conditions and reputed to have a role in the treatment of new growths.

Laryngitis

Acute or chronic infection or irritation of the laryngeal chords, with hoarseness, irritation and loss of voice. The condition may be psychological in origin with chord-paralysis until the underlying problem is resolved.

Causticum, Hepar Sulph, Aconite, Dulcamara. Chronic cases need careful diagnosis of the underlying causes. Others to consider are *Sulphur, Graphites, Arum. Triph.*

Lassitude

The common condition of exhaustion with disinterest. The causes are many and include depression, anaemia, post-convalescence, fatigue from poor work and commuting conditions. Chronic infection anywhere in the body, stress, poor diet or fasting. Also before an acute physical illness has fully declared itself.

REMEDIES
Sepia, Arnica, Nux Moschata, Kali Phos., Ferrum Phos.

Laterality of the remedies

The predisposition of certain remedies to act more strongly and effectively on one side of the body than on the other.
Right-sided remedies include
Lycopodium, Iris Versic, Kalmia, Comocladia.
Left-sided remedies include
Kreosotum, Lachesis, Eunonymus, Kali Carb. Rhus Tox.

Latrodectus Mactans (Black Widow Spider)

One of the most important spider remedies using the tincture of the whole insect. Introduced to homoepathy by Tafel and Jones. Its main indications are angina of effort, chest pain radiating down the arms, collapse and shock. There is a tendency to haemorrhage.

Laurocerasus (the common Cherry Laurel)

The fresh leaves contain prussic acid which give an indication of its potential toxicity in the undiluted state. Chill, cyanosis, convulsions, collapse and lack of vital reaction. Cough is characteristic with shortness of breath, clubbing of finger tips, cyanotic blueness as occurs in certain cardiac or chronic lung problems. The cough is typically dry, spasmodic and irritating. The overall condition is one of weakness and near-collapse, the reserves minimal.

Law of Homoeopathic Cure

This is the basic law of the similitudes whereby any natural substance able to create a physiological or psychological disturbance when taken, by a healthy person, can cure similar symptoms in a sick person. It is traditionally summarised in latin by *Similia Similibus Curentur,* or 'let like be treated by like'.

Laxatives

The amount of senna pods and other laxatives consumed by an average English family can be considerable. There is a desperate bid to stimulate natural peristalsis in a sluggish alimentary tract poisoned by over-refined foods, lack of exercise and roughage — made lazy by synthetic bowel stimulants. Often regular bowel-habits and training have been absent for many years and causes both discomfort and anxiety. When used over a prolonged period, laxatives are undesirable and should be replaced by bran, particularly using foods rich in natural vegetable roughage. The avoidance of aluminium utensils in the kitchen is also basic. The appropriate homoeopathic remedy for the type of constipation should be taken until normal bowel action has been re-established and then stopped. In general far too much energy and anxiety is centred around the problem, especially in the elderly and it should be allowed to resolve naturally without undue panic or urgency.
REMEDIES include
Alumina, Bryonia, Nux. Vom., Opium.

Lay Homoeopathy

The practise of homoeopathy by non-medically trained practioners. This occurs now in several countries including the U.K. although strictly outlawed in others as illegal medical practise. Training varies from a brief correspondence course to a three-year training and opinions vary considerably as to the advisability of the non-medical homoeopath. The B.M.A. is setting up a working party and inquiry (1983) to study alternative medicine and to consider a possible Royal Commission as now over a quarter of qualified general practitioners in this country have had some experience of either receiving or prescribing alternatives like homoeopathy. In many cases where treatment is sought, the problem is not so much one of prescribing but rather

138

of making a diagnosis. Homoeopathy should not just be regarded as a panacea cure-for-all or the inevitable prescription. Many cases require a surgical approach or sometimes a combination of tretments including conventional ones and the antibiotic where vital energy is exhausted or non-existant. The needs of the patient must at all times come before any necessity to prescribe, to treat or prove a principle. There is a lot of confusion in the public's mind concerning lay practise and the lay 'doctor' can undoubtedly be in some instances a nuisance even a danger because of diagnostic incompetence, inexperience and lack of training. The lay practitioner must know his limitations and always work in close contact with a trained medical qualified practitioner to refer cases when in doubt. All qualified homoeopathic physicians are fully trained medical doctors. In all cases diagnosis must be made at a proper pathological or disease-level as well as a homoeopathic one to ensure the patient's best interests. In certain countries and situations, particularly the missionary one, homoeopathy by the lay practitioner can be of enormous value and support a local population and health-programme, particularly when working closely with the medical team. Its validity in other circumstances is often doubtful, the dangers for the patient can often outweigh the usefulness. Certainly a well-experienced lay-practitioner working in close contact with a doctor and part of a team can be of enormous value to a busy practise when no other homoeopath is available. All too often this does not happen and the patient is left in doubt as to whom is his true 'doctor' and where to go for emergency help. A lay practitioner working in isolation with all the dangers of assumption and inadequate training can be a recipe for disaster. But a doctor with rigid prescribing attitudes, refusing to take an overall or in-depth appraisal of the patient, unwilling to ever consider an alternative approach to a problem, is scarcely better.

Ledum (marsh tea, wild rosemary)

An important first-aid remedy which has anti-parasitic action. Weakness and coldness are typically present with lowered resistance. It is especially recommended for puncture wounds due to animal or insect bites as from a cat, monkey, needle-injury, or bee or wasp sting. Redness with swelling and throbbing pain is an indication with chill and cold accompanying inflammation or

139

fever. In spite of general chillyness they are always worse for the heat of the bed. (*Pulsatilla*).

Legs — heavy

Caused by poor circulation from leg-swelling and swollen ankles. The underlying cause is usually associated with varicose veins, infection, or sometimes the cause is heart or kidney malfunctioning. In all cases the circulation is sluggish, fluid accumulates in the leg tissues causing discomfort.

REMEDIES
Natrum Mur, Apis, Sulphur, Lachesis, Rhus Tox, Pulsatilla, Carbo Veg, Alumina, Berberis.

Lehrmann, M.D. (-   )

One of the early homoeopathic physicians who first introduced and developed high potency prescribing.

Leucorrhoea

The condition of white or clear discharge from the vagina often associated with irritation and frequently offensive. Causes are variable but include cervical ulceration, general fatigue and lack of reserves. Infection can produce a thick purulent discharge.

REMEDIES
Calcarea, Graphites, Kali Carb, Sulphur, Pulsatilla, Sepia.

Libido

The innate sexual and ultimately vital energy of the individual. Its level of expression reaches a peak in adolescence but it varies throughout life according to many complex factors including psychological ones. The general level of health is reflected in healthy libido. Absence or lack of libido can occur in conditions of infection, deficiency, the contraceptive "pill", fatigue. In all cases libido has a natural rhythm which varies with each individual and this must be understood by both members of a relationship in order to avoid misunderstanding and needless anxiety.

REMEDIES
For lack of libido consider *Kali Iod, Selenium, Onosmodium.*
For excess libido consider *Platina, Belladonna, Murex.*

Lilienthal, Samuel. M.D. (1815–1891)

The American homoeopathic physician born in Munich who settled and qualified in New York becoming physician to the U.S. homoeopathic dispensary and professor of the New York homoeopathic medical college and hospital for women for 20 years. Editor of the *North American Journal of Homoeopathy* (1870–85). Editor of the New York *Journal of Homoeopathy* (1874).

His major writings include:
1876 *Treatise of diseases of the skin*
1878 *Homoeopathic therapeutics*
1886 *Works on the materia medica*
1886 *Hereditary insanity*
1887 *Aetiology of tuberculosis.*

Lilium Tig. (the Tiger Lily)

Tincture of the fresh plant and flowers, proved by Payne and Dunham. The remedy has a powerful action on the emotions especially where there is restless depression or irritability. Basic make-up is often the religious or 'do-gooder'. Pelvic symptoms with a bloated sensation, pains of 'bearing down' type (*Sepia*) and offensive brownish leucorrhoea Angina pectoris. All symptoms are worse for consolation (*Nat. Mur.*).

Lipoma

The small common fatty tumour — soft and mobile which occurs in the skin at any age and for no obvious cause. They sometimes cause pain and discomfort apart from being unsightly, stretching superficial nerves in the area.
REMEDIES
Graphites, Sulphur, Pulsatilla.

Lippe Dr Adolphus (1812–1888)

The early homoeopathic researcher and practitioner who first developed the C.M. potency in the U.S.
His major works include
Key to the Materia Medica;
Textbook of Materia Medica;
What is Homoeopathy?

141

Lips cracked

The common winter condition associated with chapping of face and hands.

REMEDIES

Arum Triph., Bryonia, Graphites, Lachesis, Sulphur, Silicea, Natrum Mur.

Locality of Symptom

This is important in the choice of remedy and may give the clue to prescribing together with the overall mental and psychological assessment. For example — pain in small localised areas on the scalp — as if a nail is being driven through the head is suggestive of *Thuja*. Pain just under the right shoulder blade or scapula indicates *Chelidonium*. Right-sided pain — *Lycopodium*.

Loneliness

This is a psychological condition which is increasingly common and similar to home-sickness often after a change of environment or even a holiday.

Eupatorium Purp. or *Kali Carb.* are of value for home-sickness.
Pulsatilla feels lonely unless constantly surrounded by people to give reassurance;
Lycopodium is lonely and insecure unless there is someone else in the house, although quite content to be in a room by themselves.

Lumbago

The common problem of low back ache or pain, often incapacitating and paralysing, following strain, as from lifting, poor posture or exposure to damp and cold.

REMEDIES

Rhus Tox, Bryonia, Nux Vomica, Berberis, Aconitum.

Luna (Lactose crystals exposed to the moon's rays)

Indicated in illnesses influenced by the phases of the moon, particularly worm infection — as threadworm, insomnia aggravated at the full moon. Certain psychological states, particularly those of lunar-excitement. Epilepsy and asthma are also often aggravated by the new moon. Where the moon plays a role in influencing or aggravating symptoms, then the remedy should be considered.

Lux, Wilhelm (1796–1849)

One of the early homoeopaths, active in research and who helped to introduce the M potency. Basically a vetinary surgeon from Leipsig, he developed his theories of Isopathy or that every contagious disease contains within itself its own cure. Using infective materials he developed the first nosodes from anthrax and small pox. Greatly criticised at the time, nosodes are now invaluable in prevention and treatment.

Lycopodium (Club Moss)

Tincture of the club-moss spores. Introduced by Hahnemann to homoeopathy, it is one of the most important of all polycrest remedies with powerful influence on emotional states of apprehension, fear and anticipatory anxiety as stage-fright, examination-fear and general insecurity. It acts strongly on the alimentary tract, especially for flatulence and indigestion. The lungs and bladder are supported and it is a valuable right-sided remedy as right-sided pneumonia. It has a general tonic effect and is indicated for enuresis and of considerable value in problems of impotency.

Lycopus (Bugle Weed)

Introduced by Hale as one of his new remedies to homoeopathy. Indicated whenever there are haemorrhagic tendencies, especially of the lungs or rectum, with shifting pains. The heart action is feeble and weak with frequent problems of palpitations and exhaustion.

Lyssin (Hydrophobinum)

The remedy prepared from saliva of the rabid-infected dog. Major indications are chronic headaches excitement of the entire nervous system, eclampsia of pregnancy, epilepsy and convulsions. Fits are worse for the sound of running water or of water being poured.

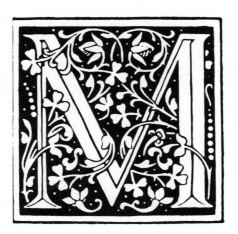

Mag. Carb (Carbonate of Magnesium)

A major constituent of the notorious Gregory's Powder of the last century — used for acidity and constipation at the time. It is indicated in dark-haired constitutions, nervous and irritable marked by exhaustion and severe prostration with over-sensitivity to the least draught of cold air or touch. At the same time they are 'touchy and sensitive'. Alimentary problems, especially colic with watery diarrhoea, vomiting and a sour taste in the mouth also suggest the remedy.

Mag. Phos (Phosphate of Magnesia)

Introduced by Schuessler to Homoeopathy and proved by Allen. One of the major remedies for cramp and spasm with shooting, changing, bouts of pain. Cold air precipitates spasm or cramp. Better for heat and warmth, for bending, doubling-up.

Often indicated in thin, anxious people, helpful for writer's cramp and where exhaustion and sweating are a feature.

Mag. Sulph. (Sulphate of Magnesia, Epsom Salts)

Collapse and prostration is severe with thirst and diarrhoea. The stools are thin and copious frequently yellow and offensive. The remedy has proved useful in the treatment of diabetes.

147

Manganum Aceticum (acetate of Manganese.)

First proved and introduced to homoeopathy by Hahnemann. Depression with irritability is characteristic. Anaemia, the skin infected with a bluish tint and chronic sore areas of ulceration failing to heal. Every part of the body is over-sensitive and tender with loss of interest in food leading to increasing weakness.

Mania

The severe psychological disturbance marked by overactivity, talkativeness, insomnia, loss of judgement and insight, violence. It usually follows a severe depressive state, although this is not always in evidence or obvious. Nash recommended a triad of remedies — *Belladonna, Hysscyamus* and *Stramonium*, depending upon the degree of violence and activity in the manic state. Hospitalisation is necessary in very severe cases.

Manic-Depressive States

The periodic psychotic illness marked by mood swings from the most profound and dangerous suicidal depressions to a 'high', excited states of optimism, agitation, insomnia and overactivity. The causes are usually obscure, but include inherited familial factors and instability in one form or other. Toxic poisons, infection, psychological shock can also act as the precipitating trigger.

REMEDIES

Natrum Mur, Sepia, Hyoscyamus, Belladonna, Stramonium.

Materia Medica

The homoeopathic materia medica is the total symptom-picture of each remedy according to proving studies, toxicology, and clinical experience. Symptoms are grouped according to major phsyiological systems of the body e.g. lungs, heart, kidneys, etc., including the modalities and other distinguishing features which combine to form a total overall picture of the remedy's action. This data is then used to match the overall symptoms of the patient forming the major homoeopathic indication to prescribe.

Mastitis

Inflammation of breast tissue often during lactation. It can also occur at any time from a blow or during a period of debility.
REMEDIES
Belladonna, Conium Mac., Phytolacca, Hepar Sulph, Merc Sol., Arnica, Aconitum.

Masturbation

Masturbation is not an illness or a disease and should not be treated as such. It is a totally normal and universal expression of sexuality. In many cases its absence may be more significant than its occurence. Only when painful or inappropriate is there a possible cause for alarm and treatment, or when it becomes part of obsessional disease. In most cases it is the natural expression of our libidinal-tides and life-force. When it causes comment or problems then the disturbance may be more in the commentator than in the other person. In general it should be regarded as 'normal', not made into an anxiety-laden 'heavy' area and a more overall loving, tolerant attitude taken. Sometimes it intrudes into adult sexual relationships and undermines it, when counselling may be needed to explore underlying causes. There are no specific remedies.

Mechanism of action of homoeopathic remedies

The exact pathway of action of the remedies is still uncertain and a matter of research. The most likely mode of action is through the immune-defensive system using the natural antibody-reactions to infection and stress. Probably the essential vital energy reaction which is characteristic of the remedies is canalised by the antigen-immune system because the steroid drugs which use the same pathway inhibit the vital response or dampen it down. We also know that many remedies can act prophylactically or preventively in illness where the remedies or appropriate nosodes are used, suggesting a specific antibody pathway. Homoeopathy acts powerfully to lessen shock and severe stress reactions of trauma and accident which is again suggestive of the same immune mechanism. Doubtless we shall see confirmation of the exact mechanism within the next few years as techniques improve further.

Medicine — the homoeopathic system of

Homoepathy is individualisation and contrasts with the allopathic method of treatment by opposites — largely based on synthetic products of the pharmaceutical industry. Homoeopathy acts in total contrast by gently supporting basic vital resistance and responses blocked by the disease-process. These vital responses are expressed by the healthy 'fighting-reaction' of the individual and are basic to health and its maintainance. The key-point of all homoeopathic medicine is the use of the 'like' or simillimum remedy which produces similar symptoms to the patient's own reactions when in its undiluted form. The single remedy, unrepeated is given as long as the patient is responding and is basic to the method. The principle of using small, serial dilutions, vitalised by succussion in the preparation of the remedy to avoid side-effects is also characteristic of homoeopathy.

Medorrhinum (Gonorrhoea Nosode)

The medorrhinum nosode is prepared from gonorrhoeal-infected material. Major symptomatology is loss of memory and a sense of impatience as if everything is happening too slowly so that impatient-hurrying and rush is common. Pain in joints is frequent, always worse in the mornings and also there is generalised tenderness, worse for touch and exhaustion. A painful tendo-achilles or ball of foot is commonly present. In general the remedy is considerably better for sea air (cp. *Natrum Mur.*).

Medusa (Jelly-fish)

Indicated mainly for skin conditions with burning irritation, redness, with blisters as in urticaria. Numbness. The whole area swollen with severe discomfort. Anxiety is marked. Useful in allergic swelling of the face, lips and eyes.

Memory Weakness

In many cases this is due to stress so that concentration and attention is impaired — the memory not given a sufficiently concentrated stimulus for recall to occur. Equally the cause may be one of degeneration, alcoholism or infection. During a convalescent period, attention is weak. After certain physical treatments as E.C.T. (electro-convulsion-therapy). In the majority of cases the cause is anxiety or stress with memory weakness heightening anxiety already present.

REMEDIES

Lycopodium, Medorrhinum, Aurum Met, Lil. Tig, Mat. Mur, Nux Vom, Kali Carb.

Menières Disease

The degenerative condition of the middle ear with deafness, tinnitus, nausea and vomiting with giddyness.

REMEDIES

Salicyl. Ac., Silicea, Lycopodium, Chininum Sulph.

Meningitis

Inflammation of the meninges or fine membrane layer covering the brain and spinal cord and conveying the cerebro-spinal circulation and nutritional cushioning fluid. Most causes are of viral type in recent years, although the bacterial form can still occur. Acute infection occurs with irritation of the whole area affected. Symptoms include severe headache, high temperature, stiffness of the neck region, confusion, irritability, fits or delirium. The patient must be treated in hospital whenever possible.

REMEDIES

Aconitum, Arsenicum, Sulphur, Hepar Sulph.

Menopause — problems of

Because of an inbalance of oestrogen/progesterone hormonal levels many distressing symptoms occur in the 40-50 year age group. Primarily a female problem but symptoms also occur in the male. Hot drenching flushes, severe day and night sweats, irritability, tearfulness, tachycardia (rapid heart beat) anxiety, irregularity or cessation of the periods and psychological lability are the major problem areas.

REMEDIES

Pulsatilla, Lachesis, Lil. Tig., Calcarea, Sulphur, Sanguinaria.

151

Mentals and Homoeopathy

The psychology of the individual and his state of mind has always been regarded as a key aspect of homoeopathic diagnosis and cure. One hundred years before Freud's genius gave us the importance of unconscious motivation and direction, Hahnemann firmly rooted homoeopathy in the psychology of the individual. The mentals or psychological aspects are always given a great deal of attention in the homoeopathic consultation — especially any loss of drive, tendency towards depression, moodyness, or flatness of feelings. Excessive lability of emotion, anything that causes a flood of tears — music, book or film, dreams, over-control, irritability and aggression or the inability to express it in any form is also important. Unreasonable fears, phobias or obsessional elements present in the make-up, the general state of confidence and mental well-being are all relevant as also the physical side and specific symptoms — either mental or physical. The mentals reflect the deepest and most important layers of personality. When a remedy is prescribed in sufficiently high potency it is often within these mental layers that a first imrovement occurs — a sense of well-being, feeling alive, no longer 'in gear' or 'driving with the brake on'. Even when there is a temporary aggravation of a physical problem at the outset of homoeopathy the mentals often show the first real improvement in attitude and confidence and this is usually maintained through any period of aggravation and initial movement towards cure.

Mercurius (Merc. Sol., Quicksilver)

Originally the ammonium nitrate salt of the metal was used by Hahnemann but in later years he used the tituration of the pure metal with superior results. This has been the practise since. Hahnemann both introduced and proved the metal as a remedy and gave a very comprehensive account of all its indications. Chillyness is common with profuse sweating. All symptoms are aggravated by both heat and cold and often worse at night. Offensive breath and sweating is marked with restlessness and tremor. Inflammation, ulceration with discharge of pus is typical together with congestion of the liver, and tenderness over the area. Parkinsonism with severe tremor is another indication.

Mercurius Corrosive (Mercuric Chloride)

This is an even more acute remedy than Mercurius, all the symptoms are most intense and violent. There are acute urinary symptoms with frequency, pain, haematuria and mucous in the urine. Urethritis with gonorrhoea or a greenish-yellow discharge of pus is a common symptom. There may be an acute throat — the tonsils ulcerated and discharging pus, or an alimentary tract infection with diarrhoea or dysentery-like symptoms.

Mercurius Cyanotus (Mercuric Cyanide)

Introduced by Beck for acute cases of diptheria. The main indications are collapse, the throat covered with a whitish-grey mucous thick coating, with rawness, difficult swalling and speech painful. In general the patient is chilly and blue due to cyanosis from lack of oxygen. It may be indicated as a prophylactic for diptheria.

Metal Remedies

It was the genius of Hahnemann that allowed the insoluble metals to be used in homoeopathy potency by grinding them into sugar of milk until a soluble substance was obtained — called trituration. The major metal remedies are *Copper (Cuprum), Selenium, Tin, (Stannium), Aluminium, Iron (Ferrum), Silver (Argentum), Gold (Aurum).*

Mezereum (Daphne Mezereum)

Tincture of the pure bark taken before the plant flowers in February. There is a burning crusty eruption over the whole scalp or face with itching eczema, ulcers and thick scabs often whitish in colour. Everywhere is a burning neuralgic-type pains. Depression is common with exhaustion and sometimes the odd but characteristic sensation of the teeth being too long. All symptoms are aggravated in the early spring when the plant is in flower. There is also aggravation from damp or cold and a dislike of being touched or examined.

153

Miasms

One of the most important and unique contributions of homoeopathy to the treatment and causation of chronic disease. Hahnemann describes in *Chronic Disease* three major pathways of hereditary constitutional disease containing not the disease itself but its blueprint or 'shadow' of the original disease. Psora was most important or the 'Itch', Sycosis is illness with a primarily gonorrhoeal root; and Syphilis is the miasmic illness having a syphilitic origin in previous generations. Hahnemann worked for many years with his colleagues on the problem of chronic disease and developed a comprehensive list of recommended remedies for each miasm. For greater detail see headings listed under the individual miasm.

Migraine

The common syndrome of periodic headache, often one-sided, commonly beginning over one eye, associated with nausea, dislike of light and brightness of any kind. Prostration, flashing lights and sometimes vomiting as the headache becomes more severe and fixed is characteristic. Migraine tends to occur in cycles with periods of several weeks free from all symptoms. It is often familial and to date there is no known pathological cause.

REMEDIES
Lycopodium (right-sided migraine), *Iris Versicolor* (right-sided), *Lachesis* (left-sided), *Kali Carb* (left-sided), *Coffea, Kalmia* (right-sided).

Milk Allergy

Although this can occur throughout life, it is most commonly seen in the young child with projectile vomiting and failure to thrive because of sensitivity to cow's milk.

REMEDY
Aethusa followed by a constitutional prescription.

Mineral Remedies

These form a large and most important group of remedies with far-reaching effects upon the patient, especially in areas of vitality, basic energy and energy-reserves as well as the internal

154

organs, alimentary tract and skin. Often insoluble, like the metals they are made into soluble solution by grinding and dilution with lactose. They include *Silicea, Phosphorus, Sulphur, Antimony.* There are various very active mineral acids for example *Fluoric Acid, Nitric Acid, Phosphoric Acid, Sulphuric Acid, Acetic Acid, Benzoic Acid, Oxalic Acid* as well as the various mineral salts as *Arsenicum Alb, Mag. Phos.* Potassium salts include *Potassium Carbonate, Sulphate* and *Bromide.* Sodium Chloride in potency as the invaluable *Natrum Mur* is another of the deepest and widest acting mineral salts.

Mixed Autumn Pollens (M.A.P.)

Tincture of three tree moulds — Mucor, Aspergillus and Penicillin. This is a most useful mixed homoeopathic preparation for hay-fever-like symptoms occuring in early autumn, particularly September, with sneezing, nasal catarrh, tightness of chest, itchy eyes and throat.

Modalities of the patient

These are the characteristic constitutional features of the patient which are quite unique and relate to environmental responses to heat, cold, damp, wind, dryness, thunder, sea-air, water, heights, time of day, time-of-season and foods. As a totality they create a sense of well-being or fatigue and aggravation of the condition. For example *Pulsatilla* and *Arg. Nit.* are both totally intolerant of heat in any form although *Pulsatilla* is at the same time chilly. In contrast *Rhus Tox, Arsenicum* and *Calcarea* all crave heat but in slightly different characteristic ways when the overall picture of each remedy is looked at in detail. It is the combination of modalities combined with the total symptom-picture which makes for the individualisation of approach and accuracy of prescribing.

Morbillinum (the measles nosode)

Usually given in the 30th potency as a prophylactic or in rare cases of acute severe measles illness. Indications would be cough, nasal and conjuctival congestion, sore throat, middle ear pain and involvement and the typical skin rash. In a very young baby it is of value when there has been exposure, particularly if the infant is especially vulnerable.

Morgan Co. (Bach)

The bowel nosode, with special action on the skin and portal circulation of the liver. Congestion is the key-note with pounding congestive headaches or migraine attacks. There is a general liverish tendency with bilious headaches, gall-stones, burning acid indigestion. Constipation is present in 95% cases. The mentals are anxiety with irritability.

Moschus (Musk Deer)

Tincture of the dried preputial secretion of the Musk deer. The major indication is a tendancy to faint easily, particularly at the least emotion with pallor and chilliness. The patient looks deathly pale in the faint as if there were no life left at all. Sweating and marble-whiteness adds to the general impression of lifelessness. It is useful in Premenstural Tension but especially it is of value in nervous tension of the hysterical make-up.

Mother-tincture (symbol used is θ)

The basic remedy in solution before dilution, sometimes after trituration when an initially insoluble mineral or metal is used. After agitation and thorough mixing, usually in a water-alcohol mixture, the mother-tincture forms the basis of the potencies. For the centisimal dilutions, one drop of tincture in 99 drops of the serial dilutant fluid is used in alcohol solution. In some cases the remedy is given as the mother tincture in drop form and not put up into potency, although prescribed according to simillimum principles. Here the remedy is needed to act at a strictly organ or tissue level only. The commonest example is *Crataegus,* taken as a heart tonic and commonly prescribed in this form as drops taken in water. Also *Phytolacca berry* for problems of obesity, *Sabal Serrulata* for prostatic problems and the remedy *Plantago.* But these are the exceptions rather than the rule in homoeopathy and for the majority of cases a potentised remedy is made up from the mother-tincture to encompass the mental side as well as the tissue level of the problem.

Muscle Pains

This is a common problem and naturally treatment varies according to symptoms and cause. When traumatic in origin with bruising, *Arnica* is indicated followed by *Bellis* and then *Ruta* for injury to muscle. If the problem is rheumatic in origin with joint swelling or weakness *Rhus Tox* is a major indicated remedy. When due to night-cramps of uncertain origin in the calf muscles give *Cuprium Aceticum*. Pain in the calf muscles on exercise may be circulatory in origin and require *Cactus*, but such symptoms are best treated under the direction of a physician. Pain associated with allergic swelling in the area may need *Urtica*.

Myxoedema

Deficiency of thyroid functioning due to simple goitre and lack of mineral Iodine in the diet. In other cases it is a complication of surgery for thyroid overactivity where excessive removal of thyroid tissue has occured. Other causes are obscure and unknown but often of a degenerative type.
REMEDIES
Thyriod 3X, Baryta Carb 6, Calcarea.
In all cases the cause of the underlying reduced functioning must be ascertained and corrected.

Murex (Purple fish)

Trituration of the fresh juice of the fish. First proved by Petroz. The remedy is indicated where there is hypersensitivity, excitement, emotional tension and hysterical tendencies, often with heightened libido. It is useful at the menopause when there are irregular periods with the formation of the clots. There is a characteristic profound dislike of being touched or examined.

157

Naevus

The common pigmented beauty spot or mole. It requires no treatment unless very generalised or widespread and should not be removed or interfered with unless in a part of the body where there is constant chronic irritation or where they have appreciably changed in shape, size, thickness or surface form. In such cases they may require removal by an experienced surgeon.
REMEDIES
Thuja, Carcinosin, Phosphorus.

Naja (the Indian Cobra Venom)

One of the most ancient of all medical remedies using tincture of the fresh cobra venom. Many of the symptoms are of a cardiac nature with burning, weight-like oppression in the chest and a slow pulse. There is cardiac collapse, the pulse slow, shortness of breath and a sensation of choking. Many symptoms are aggravated by lying down and are usually left-sided. Depression is the commonest mental state.

Napthalinum (Napthalene)

Indicated for drowsy, confused states as high toxic infected states with delirium. Also recommended for hay fever, whooping cough and threadworms.

161

Nasal Catarrh

The common often seasonal problem of inflammation and thickening of the nasal lining secretory layer or mucosa. There is congestion with discharge and infection. Catarrh may be allergic in origin and part of hay-fever particularly when it occurs in early June or July. The allergic response to the grass pollens causes irritation of the mucosal layer which accounts for the severe itching and watery discharge. A similar condition occurs in the autumn with allergy to late-summer tree moulds. Other allergic substances are house-dust, foods, mites and a variety of substances, as animal hair, all of which may provoke an allergic response. In others air conditioning, over-heating, lack of humidity in the office causes irritation and a chronic condition aggravated by poor quality canteen-food, over-rich in milky-carbohydrates, refined starches and sugars.

The common winter cold is perhaps the commonest cause of all with nose, throat and eyes affected by the inflammation and discharging profusely. The temperature is high whilst vitality and strength are at zero because of toxicity from the infection.

REMEDIES

Kali Carb, Mixed pollens, M.A.P., Kali Bic, Gelsemium, Allium Cepa.

Nash, E. R., M.D. (1838-   )

One of the early American influential homoeopathic workers. His best known writing is *'Leaders in Homoeopathic Therapeutics'* (1898). Other writings include *Leaders for the use of Sulphur, The Testimony of the Clinic, How to take the case, Leaders in Typhoid Fever, Regional Leaders.*

Natrum Carb. (Sodium Carb or the common 'soda')

First proved by Hahnemann and recommended for chronic psora conditions with severe skin problems of irritation, soreness, dry chapped burning hands and face without discharge. There is catarrh and a sore throat, the alimentary tract congested and causing problems of chronic indigestion. A similar problem occurs in the uterine area where congestion causes leucorrhoea. The predominant mood is depression and irritation with

162

twitching and exhaustion. All the chronic problems are worsened by heat, music and effort.

Natrum Phosphoricum (Phosphate of sodium)

Introduced first by Schuessler as a tissue-salt. A remedy for chronic problems of indigestion with sourness of taste or vomiting from excess milk in the diet. Lactic acid is generally in excess. The tongue is covered with a thick, sour-smelling coating and the diarrhoea is of a similar yellowish colour. Acidity, colic, flatulence and discomfort is marked. Depression with irritability is the main mental attitude with general misery and dissatisfaction.

Natrum Sulph (Sodium Sulphate)

Formerly Glauber's Salt and introduced to homoeopathy by Schluessler and Grauvogl. Primarily it is a remedy for sycotic conditions where the symptoms are in the pancreatic bile duct regions which are not functioning effectively. There is chronic indigestion, constipation, colic — the whole intestinal region tender and sluggish. Bladder problems are common with frequency, bed-wetting, constipation. All symptoms are worse for damp or cold, tight clothing, music, better for cold dry weather and fresh air.

Natrum Mur (Sodium Chloride or common salt)

One of the most valuable and important of all the polycrests and well-documented by Compton-Burnett. Mental symptoms are depression with irritability, tearfulness — worse for consolation and company is characteristic. The remedy acts strongly on kidney functioning and has an important role to play in fluid and water balance. Retention both mental and physical is a common feature and indication for the remedy — fluid accumulating in the soft tissues of the body, especially the face, lower eyelids, which are puffy and bloated as the body generally. There is always chillyness and profound exhaustion with typical craving for excess salt in the diet. Chronic digestive problems are due to sluggish congestion. Also diarrhoea and Cataract. Most patients are either better or aggravated by sea air. (*Medorrhinum*).

Nausea

The sensation of general malise, sweating and weakness with an overwhelming desire to vomit. The condition may be provoked by a gastric upset following a dietary indiscretion or acute infection. It is also common in the early months of pregnancy. Many cases are psychological in origin and provides an exit from a threatening overwhelming situation. The underlying causes must be thoroughly diagnosed and investigated.

REMEDIES

Nux Vom, Natrum Mur, Ipecac., Arg. Nit., Pulsatilla, Cocculus.

Neatby, Edwin A. (1858–1933)

The London Homoeopath and nephew of Thomas Neatby, working in general practise with his uncle in Hampstead before specialising in gynaecology. Eventually physician for diseases of women at the London Homoeopathic Hospital in 1922. President of the British Homoeopathic Society in 1897 and 1919; Founder of the Missionary School in 1903 and later dean, establishing its present premises at 2, Powis Place. He was responsible for much of the schools appeal and success. Author of many articles in the homoeopathic journals.

Major writings include:

A manuel of Tropical Medicine and hygiene, (written with Thomas Miller Neatby);

A manual of homoeotherapeutics (written with T. Stonham).

Neatby, Thomas Miller. M.D. (–   )

One of the early homoeopathic physicians of the century, physician to the London Homoeopathic Hospital and the Missionary School. He was conservative in his approach, a pupil and active supporter of Hughes and his pathological approach and logic. He opposed the then new American ideas of high, single remedy prescriptions and potencies. He was co-author of *A Handbook of Tropical Medicine and Hygiene* with his nephew Edwin Neatby.

Neck pain and stiffness

The common problem of pain and aching discomfort in the neck area. The cause is variable — from a simple traumatic cause with bruising and spasm, or exposure to draught with chill and tension in local muscles of the area or tenderness and stiffness. Muscular rheumatism is a more recurrent problem, related to damp or sudden climatic changes, aggravated by age and poor health generally. Neck pain may also come from a nearby vertebral cause where arthritis or displacement, infection, or any localised condition causes pressure or irritation. The condition may also be acute or chronic. Not uncommonly it is psychological in origin, the tension and pain due to underlying anxiety and reflecting deeper problems. If more hysterical in type, symptoms can be incapacitating with a dramatic, attention-seeking element which defies all attempts at either diagnosis or cure.

REMEDIES
Rhus Tox, Causticum, Aconitum, Arnica, Natrum Mur, Sulphur.

Nephritis

Strictly pyelonephritis with infection of the kidney tissue. Common in either sex but especially the female when it may be recurrent with bouts of severe loin pain, tenderness, high temperature and a variety of urinary symptoms. It is common in pregnancy. The cause is a bacterial infection; either blood-transmitted or ascending via the ureters from an infected bladder (cystitis). The illness must be thoroughly diagnosed and treated to avoid a chronic condition with all the risks of renal impairment and circulatory complications.

REMEDIES
Hepar Sulph., Mercurius, Aconitum, Sycotic Co, Causticum, Cantharis, Berberis.

Nervous Illness

The commonest problem seen in our stress-laden society. It is prsent at all ages in all countries and involves every ethnic group. Nervousness reflects underlying emotional tension, stress, lack of confidence, uncertainty and fear. It is seen from childhood to old age and feeds on natural fears, uncertainties and anxieties concerned with war, social tensions and any lack of physical or spiritual health and faith. Much of the present emotional stress is related to the enormous psychological pressures that are placed on all of us — to be different, to live up to some media-ideal with changes in speed, tempo, rhythm and life-patterns. Many are ill-prepared for such pressures and quite unable to adapt or adjust — from lack of training and education as to the best attitude and approach to take. Indeed there is no formal attention or education given to this area because of the common emphasis on examination success rather than the broader needs of the individual and problem-solving in life as well as in the classroom. Flexibility, alternative solutions, adjustment to life's changes and problems are largely ignored and denied within our educational system to the personal loss of the individual. Homoeopathy can help enormously in some areas, supporting the underlying psychology. But in all cases, a natural rhythm and overall mature approach to life, change and challenge is essential and must be fostered and supported throughout life.

REMEDIES
Nux Vom, Natrum Mur, Gelsemium, Ignatia, Sulphur, Arsenicum, Lycopodium.

Neuralgia

Pain — not necessarily psychological and often caused by underlying physical local irritation as with dental neuralgia. The cause is not always apparent. There is irritation of nerves in the affected area and mechanical factors, infection, draughts and chill all play a part in the problem. Pain may be severe and chronic.

REMEDIES
Coffea, Kalmia, Chamomilla, Nux. Vom, Sulphur, Spigelia, Rhus Tox.

Neurosis

The common psychological condition where nervous symptoms due to stress intrude into everyday life and undermine relation-ships. Efficiency, concentration, joy, peace of mind — either at work or in home-relationships are absent, limited or sporadic. Common symptoms are physical ones with recurrent colds, pains, chronic back-ache or fatigue. More obvious psychological symptoms are dpression, hysteria, tearfulness and collapse.

Phobias or obsessions may occur but not invariably. Often there is an inability to either build or maintain personal relationships with loneliness, self-imposed isolation and a sense of futility. Underlying causes need to be explored, understood, verbalised, discussed and shared. There is no magic — and distorted assumptions or viewpoints about the motivations of others need to be replaced by more giving, interest, sharing and caring. In many cases, self-interest and self-protection has become more important than relationships and other people.

REMEDIES

These include the specific constitional prescription. For specifics see section — *Nervousness*.

Nitric Acid (Aqua Fortis)

A valuable recommended remedy. There is depression in an anxious, usually thin and dark-complexioned person with skin problems especially around the junction-areas of skin and mucous membrane as the corners of the mouth or the ears or anal area. Typical symptoms are fissure or fistula with cutting, stich-like pains, sharp and sudden, a tendency to haemorrhage from any exposed fissure or ulcer. These areas are extremely tender and are common inside the mouth and on the tongue as ulcers, usually worse for acid fruits and certain wines.

Also indicated for pneumonia, bronchitis, diarrhoea with blood in the stools as typhus fever. Severe pain on opening the bowels and attempting to pass a motion. The urine has a characteristic horse-like odour.

Nosode

The potentised homoeopathic remedy prepared from diseased pathological tissue used to prevent or treat the associated disease of the tissue material. First introduced by Lux in the face of much controversy, it has found a place in homoeopathy which has proved to be of enormous value and without risk to the patient. It is of particular-use in chronic conditions. In general the nosode should not be repeated for 6 months after the initial prescription. Examples include *Morbillinum,* (measles) *Varicellinum* (chicken pox), *Tub Bov* (Tuberculosis), *Anthracinum,* (Anthrax), *Medorrhinum* (gonorrhoea), *Pertussin* (whooping cough), bowel nosdes of Bach and Paterson.

Nux Moschata (Nutmeg)

The tincture is made from the seeds. Mental symptoms of exhaustion, fatigue and collapse are marked sometimes with excitement and unreality. There is a sense of confusion, or having a dual or double personality. The condition resembles drunken stupor with weakness, chill, loss of memory and fainting. Thirst is absent (compare *Apis, Pulsatilla*).

Nux Vomica (the Poison Nut)

Tincture of the seed. One of the most important of all the polycrests especially where there are spasms of irritability, convulsions and fits of pain, temper or colic. It is especially indicated for the over-stretched executive who must at all costs keep everything 'buttoned-up' and buried inside. Extreme spasms of 'flare-up', uncontrollable sensitivity and excitability are characteristic signs for the remedy. It is especially useful for the zealous passionate types of temperament where everything is taken to heart, and they too quickly become involved — usually with what they see as the plight of the underdog. There is excessive emotion and feeling for the least thing or discussion — flaring-up and boiling-over with outbursts and just as quickly calming down again and apologetic. The physical make-up is of the thin 'Cassius' type — deep, unhappy, always thinking and scheming, full of resentments, woe and concern. Constipation is frequent and painful, the stools kept in and retained — much as the personality. Haemorrhoids, chronic gastritis, indigestion, peptic ulcer, flatulence and heatburn are common. They tend to be chilly and aggravated from any interference with sleep patterns.

Obesity

The disease of excess weight seen in all ages but particularly prevalent in the middle years and 40-year age group. It is associated with hormonal or psychological inbalance at a time when very profound physiological changes are occuring as well as the extra stress of the 'mid-life' depressive crisis. Over the years, the tendency has usually been to try and cope or control problems at whatever level by snacking to calm themselves in the face of the unknown — resorting to food — the familiar. Apart from other contrived and rarer mannerisms as tics and facial gestures — often beyond conscious control, the commonest familiar reassurance-mechanism is undoubtedly food and creature-comfort. Constantly repeating this reassuring comforting experience of eating throughout the day, together with lack of exercise, quickly contributes to body weight and size, adding to any depression. Organic causes include diabetes, Addison's disease, thyroid disorders especially Myxoedema and the side-effects of steroid drugs. Cardiac or renal failure with water retention are rarer contributory causes. Remedies must at all times take into account the underlying causes as well as the overall psychological and physical picture.

REMEDIES

Calcarea, Kali Carb, Phytolacca Berry, Thyroidinum Crataegus, Hammamelis, Apis.

Obsessional Neurosis

The psychological disorder where the major emphasis is control of self and others by rigid infantile magical thinking, psychological dogma and ritual. The aim of the obsessional defence, extensively described by Freud, is to prevent the buffettings and vicissitudes of fate — of life really, from imposing themselves upon the obsessional, catching him unawares, 'off-guard' so to speak so that he feels unprepared and in danger of being shown-up as a failure. Pride is strong in the make-up and failure a terrifying nightmare. There is a multitude of fears and threats in every area of life imaginable. All the rituals of avoiding cracks in the pavement, ladders, double-checking doors and gas-taps is to prevent being caught-out so to speak with his 'pants down'. This gives a clue to the infantile nature of its origins and the terror of being found defenseless and in a state of panic.
REMEDIES
Arg. Nit, Platina, Natrum Mur, Lycopodium, Gelsemium.

Ocimum Canum (Alfavaca)

Introduced to homoeopathy by Mure. A major remedy for right-sided renal colic where there is a red sandy deposit in the urine. Vomiting and collapse from renal colic. Kidney stones, cystitis with infection. Restlessness. Musk odour to the urine.

Oedema

Excess of fluid in the tissues of any part of the body including the heart (pericardial oedema), lungs (pulmonary oedema), abdominal cavity (peritoneal oedema), limbs — the common ankle oedema, throat or soft palate (angioneurotic oedema). The most frequent type is oedema of the lower limb with ankle swelling, pitting on pressure, swelling of the feet, ankles and legs. Symptoms are better for rest and in the mornings, worse for standing or fatigue. The legs feel heavy, like lead with pain, discomfort and slowness because of fluid retention. With the possible exception of lower limb oedema, all forms need treatment by a physician, often in hospital. Leg oedema may be caused by many factors including cardiac weakness or heart failure and kidney disease but most commonly poor circulation from varicose veins. Other causes of leg swelling and oedema are phlebitis, local trauma, blockage of the lymphatic circulation, allergy and infection. Careful diagnosis and a detailed history is essential to exclude an obstructive or surgical condition which needs early referral for treatment. If there is a surgical condition causing blockage, this must be dealt with by surgical correction because mechanical interference to flow and drainage cannot usually be relieved by homoeopathy.

REMEDIES

Pulsatilla, Calcarea, Natrum Mur, Apis, Hammamelis, Sulphur, Alumina.

Oleander (Rose Laurel)

Tincture of the leaves, first proved by Hahnemann. There is anxiety with faintness. Primarily this is a cardiac remedy with problems of severe palpitations, weakness, collapse and dizzyness. Vertigo, diarrhoea, gastro-enteritis, are common. The skin is often raw, with rough chapping and soreness. Depression is the major emotional mood.

Onosmodium (False Gromwell)

Tincture of the fresh plant, first proved by Green in 1887. There is tension with irritability, the person impatient, in a hurry unable to ever relax as time passes so very slowly (*Medorrhinum*). Judgement and concentration are poor with accident proneness (*Kali Carb*) Muscular weakness, wasting of muscles, incoordination, long-sightedness of the elderly, blurred double vision, eye strain, headaches, vertigo are characteristic.

Operations — the use of homoeopathy in surgical procedures

It is advisable to take *Arnica 30* both before and after an operation in order to reduce shock, swelling and bruising and to cut down the risk of haemorrhage. It also tends to shorten the period of convalescent recovery. Usually one dose pre-operatively and two doses afterwards is sufficient. When there is major surgery, involving a large incision and post-operative pain, use *Staphisagria 6* for pain after *Arnica.*

For pre-operative fear and anxiety use *Arg. Nit. 200*, in three equal doses, preferably in powder form and during the 48 hour period preceding the operation. For post-operative chest conditions with cough, aching pain and a dry irritating need to constantly clear the throat and chest — worse for the least jarring movement or draught of cold air, give *Byronia 6* three times daily until the symptoms have stopped. If inflammation develops post-operatively with burning red streaks along an arm or limb, tender to the least pressure and with temperature use *Belladonna 6* three times daily and let the physician advise as to other treatment necessary. In all cases the correct homoeopathic prescription makes the paient more comfortable and speeds the recovery time. Always stop the remedies as soon as the patient is better and free from symptoms. Do not continue them needlessly.

Opium (Papaver Somniferum)

Tincture of the unripe poppy capsule. The main indications and symptoms are those of acute cerebral catastrophe or 'stroke', with loss of consciousness, coma, pin-point fixed pupils and immobility. The face is bloated with a purple cyanotic hue and there may be noisy vomiting or the breathing slow and laboured and noisy. Also for drowsyness, confusion, falling-about with unsteadyness or delirium. Constipation is absolute with flatus passed but lack of reaction in all areas generally including to pain. Snoring.

Orchitis

Inflammation of the testicle. Commonly associated with infection by the mumps virus either in childhood or the adult. The latter causes a more severe reaction and illness, sometimes leading to sterility. In some cases the origin is unknown, due to trauma or other infective agents. There is pain, swelling and discomfort.
REMEDIES
Pulsatilla, Clematis, Hamamelis, Rhododendron, Spongia.

Organic Illness

As opposed to emotional or psychological illness, there is pathology or disease in an organ or part of the body, creating interference with normal functioning leading to blockage and interference with the physiology of the part affected and sometimes of the surrounding area. The illness may also affect the central nervous system and cause interference with the normal psychological state and the symptoms themselves provoke reactions of fear and anxiety because they are unfamiliar, not understood or seem illogical. An organic illness may or may not be ammenable to homoeopathic treatment, depending upon the degree of obstruction and interference with normal functioning. A cyst or goitre may put pressure on surrounding tissues or underlying passageways — perhaps the oesophagus so that there are problems of swallowing in addition to interference with thyroid functioning and surgery required to relieve the obstruction — whatever homoeopathic treatment is given. In general homoeopathy works well in organic illness provided that the remedy is correctly prescribed according to overall symptoms. There is often correction of underlying disease in the area affected provided that it is not chronic or obstructive and that there is sufficient vital energy present. As with all illness, an overal total evaluation of the patient, the symptoms and pathology must be considered. A surgical opinion is advisable in all cases, but especially where severe scarring or obstruction undermines the ability of the homoeopathy remedy to function fully.

Organon — of Hahnemann

The Organon of the Rational System of Medicine — the title taken from Aristotle as the instrument of all reasoning. First published in Leipzig in 1810, it is the most important book published by Hahnemann and sets out the whole of his philosophy of homoeopathy and its rules of application to the patient, laws of similitude and cure. The book was well received by homoeopaths the world over and has become a classic. There are six editions known of which the last edition is the most important because of the footnotes and appendices. The Organon deserves a place on the bookshelf of every serious student of homoeopathy.

Ornithogalum Umbellatum (Star of Bethlem)

Tincture of the fresh plant. Indicated for chronic digestive problems, burning pain with distention, flatulence and peptic ulceration. Especially the upper abdominal area is blown-up as if inflated — a short time after eating the smallest meal. Vomiting and heartburn are common. The predominant mood is of depression and irritability.

Ortega, Proceso S., M.D. (1919-   )

The emminent contemporary Mexican homoeopath and teacher. Founder of the Mexican teaching academy for the expansion of homoeopathic principles — *Homoeopatia de Dedico*, he has been an active teacher and physician within the International League for the past 20 years. Also director of the Mexican Journal *La homoeopatia en el Mundo*, Vice-president of the International League. In the last two international congresses, (1981/82) his group has presented papers on the chronic miasms.

Osteoporosis

Decalcification or thinning of bone with increased liability to fractures. It is a common condition of the elderly — the bones on X-ray almost transparent from loss of calcium. It may also occur after prolonged drug abuse or indiscriminate vitamin thereapy over a prolonged period.

REMEDIES
Calc. Phos., Nat. Mur, Baryta Car., Symphytum.

Otitis Media

Acute inflammation of the middle ear, with severe pain, discharge of pus or mucous, especially when the drum has burst from internal pressure on the membrane. The temperature is high, the patient restless, at times toxic. It can sometimes be a most distressing and recurrent illness of childhood.

REMEDIES
Belladonna, Ferrum Phos, Pulsatilla, Hepar Sulph., Mercurius, Sulphur.

Ovarian Problems

For ovarian cyst consider *Apis 6* when the cyst is right-sided with burning, stinging pains. *Lachesis* is more indicated for left-sided cyst and pains. A surgical opinion is essential.

For ovarian pain generally, not related to cystic conditions, but more to inflammation and hormonal disfunction use *Apis* or *Belladonna.* For pain at ovulation time consider *Colocynth, Sabina, Naja.*

Oxalic Acid (Sorrel Acid)

Indicated for painful conditions particularly of the rheumatoid type. Most symptoms are left-sided but can occur in any part of the body. There are agonising, sharp severe pains worse from thinking or worrying about the condition. Exhaustion, weakness and collapse with coldness and shock is characteristic. Vomiting of blood may occur and there is a general bleeding tendency with small red spots or petechiae from minute haemorrhages under the skin. In some cases the condition procedes to one of excitation or fits but in general exhaustion and prostration dominates the picture.

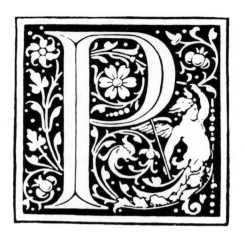

Paeonia (Paeony)

Tincture of the fresh root. This is a remedy for circulatory irregularities with profuse hot-flushes, sweats, blushing of face, trunk and head. The anus is a problem area with splinter-like pains from anal fissure, fistula or haemorrhoids. Bed sores, itching and irritation is marked and all symptoms are worse for movement of any kind. Major mental symptoms are severe restlessness or fearfulness with nightmares. Rest is the major factor to relieve symptoms and walking or movement makes them worse.

Pain

Perhaps the most distressing of all human suffering. It varies very considerably both in degree and character, also frequency, site, time of onset, aggravating factors, duration and causation.
REMEDIES
Arnica where the pain has a bruised-like quality;
Aconite — severe acute pain with restlessness and marked fear;
Arsenicum — pain is acute and burning with severe agitation;
Bryonia — the pain worse for the least movement or jarring;
Belladonna — the pain red-hot, worse for touch but better for local pressure on the affected part;
Rhus Tox — pain relieved by heat and movement generally;
Colocynth — severe colicy pain, better for doubling-up,
Nitric Acid — pains are splinter-like and sharp or burning;

181

Staphisagria — the pain is sharp, tearing, often post-operational with a marked feeling of resentment.
Nux Vom. — pain is sporadic, cramping with anger and marked irritability,
Glonoin — the pain is throbbing and beating,
Cactus — vice-like and cramping pains.

Palpitations

The common heightened awareness of the heart's action, usually with increased rapidity of heart-beat. Causes vary with shock or emotional stress. Most common symptoms come on during the day or night also at rest. there is additional psychological tension because of fear of heart disease. Excess of tea or coffee throughout the day causes similar quickening of the heart rate. Other causes are degeneration or blockage of the conducting pathways and various metabolic diseases including an over-active thyroid.
REMEDIES
Spigelia, Crataegus, Naja, Nux Vom.

Pancreatitis

The acute inflammation of the pancreas organ from infective causes usually. Symptoms are of the most severe abdominal pain, cramping and unbearable, with collapse and shock. Most cases need urgent hospitalisation and sometimes surgery.
REMEDIES
Aconitum, Iris, Iodium, Atropine, Kali Hydriod.

Paracelsus (1490–1541)

The philosopher and forerunner of Hahnemann who found a specific relationship between certain plant and mineral remedies and symptoms of disease. He described the Simillimum principle and advocated treatment of 'like by like' — able to effect impressive cures by these principles. Generally he is regarded as an innovator and a man far in advance of his time.

Paralysis

The cause may be either acute and sudden as from a stroke due to a cerebral thrombosis, raised blood pressure or haemorrhage. Infection as poliomyelitis, arterioschlerosis, trauma — as when a nerve is severed or multiple schlerosis are some of the commonest causes. The condition may be variable and transient in early phases of the condition. More chronic causes include degenerative disease — sometimes hereditary or of unknown causation like Motor Neurone Disease.

REMEDIES

Arnica for shock,
Veratrum Alb for severe collapse with shock and pallor,
Opium for stroke paralysis and unconsciousness,
Spartium for raised blood pressure,
Natrum Mur for Multiple Schlerosis,
Phosphorus for degenerative condition,
Paris for left-sided paralysis.

Pareira (Virgin Vine)

Tincture of the fresh root, proved by Fox. The main site of action is the urinary tract with severe cystitis, urgency, burning pains, stranguary (severe pain at the end of the passage of water). Urinary retention, Urethritis, with dysuria (pain on the passage of passing water). Prostate problems are also an indication.

Paris Quadrifolia (One Berry)

Tincture of the whole fruiting plant, proved by Hahnemann. It acts on mucous membrane, especially of the eyes giving conjunctivitis with pain and an odd sensation of the eyeballs protruding as in thyroid disease. It is mainly a left-sided remedy. Offensive diarrhoea, the mind restless, irritable, overactive and talkative (*Lachesis*).

Parkinsonism (Paralysis Agitans)

The chronic degenerative nervous condition, usually of the elderly with fine tremor, pill-rolling movement of thumbs and an associated increase of joint-stiffness and resistance to movement. The body is slow in motion, functioning and speech with thinking and responses generally retarded. Response to homoeopathy is often unsatisfactory where there is severe degeneration of major conducting pathways.

REMEDIES

Baryta Carb., Phosphorus, Zinc. Met., Arsenicum, Nux. Vom.

Parotidinum (the mumps nosode)

The remedy made from infected parotid glandular tissue and often used prophylactically in the 30th potency. Of especial value when there are vulnerable adults in contact with the disease who have not been previously affected and therefore have no immunity. The illness is mainly severe in the adult and it can be used to advantage in the 30 or 200c potency when there are complications as high temperatures, orchitis, meningitis.

Pashero, Tomas Pablo, M.D. (1904–   )

The eminent contemporary Buonos Ares homoeopath and co-founder of the Argentinian Homoeopathic Medical Association since 1934. An authority on the importance of the Organon in Homoeopathic literature as also the importance of psychological factors and the mentals in homoeopathy. He has contributed many important papers in this field at International Congresses. *The Mental Symptoms in Homoeopathy* (1975) is of especial importance.

Passiflora Incarnata (Passion flower)

Introduced by Hale to homoeopathy. A useful remedy for spasmodic conditions with violent contractions. Tetanus, epilepsy, pureperal convulsions, asthma, whooping cough. Indicated in manic excitement and delirium tremens.

Paterson, Elizabeth. M.D. (1907–1963)

Wife and co-worker of John Paterson, who did so much to establish the importance of the bowel nosodes in prescribing. A Glsgow graduate, she practised homoeopathy with her husband and they spent most of their lives working and teaching in Glasgow. Working with Dishington and Wheeler, influenced by Bach, they formed the key workers who separated the two major

184

Morgan strains of Gaertner and Sycotico with their major characteristics and indications.

Her individual writings include:

1935 *Chronic miasms and prescribing*
1941 *Nuitrition*
1959 *A survey of the nosodes*

Paterson, John. M.D. (–1954)

The emminent Glasgow homoeopathic teacher and researcher. President of the International League and President of the Homoeopathic faculty. His general papers include — *Hahnemann's doctrine of Psora, The Homoeopathic treatment of skin diseases.* He followed Dishington as physician at the Glasgow children's hospital Mount Vernon and continued his pioneering work. Together with his wife Elizabeth, they established the clinical indications for such important bowel nosodes as Dysenter Co, Morgan, Gaertner and Sycotic Co.

This entirely new group of remedies, developed from the non-lactose fermenting bacteria, normally present in the bowel are of enormous clinical importance and have widely extended the range and scope of the homoeopathic pharmacy.

Pertussin (Coqueluchin)

The nosode of the whooping cough virus, used very effectively in the prevention and treatment of disease without the risks of conventional vaccine treatment to the nervous system. It is often given from the 6th month onwards.

Petroleum (Coal Oil)

Trituration of rectified oil. First proved by Hahemann, it is one of his major anti-psora remedies and primarily indicated for skin symptoms where there is chronic eczema with soreness and redness with itching. Deep red cracks are common. The mood is one of peevish irritability — flaring-up into bursts of anger and rage. Nausea, headaches in the occiput area are characteristic and all symptoms are aggravated by cold or movement.

Petroselinum (Parsley)

Tincture of the fresh plant. First proved by Bethmann it acts mainly on the urinary system with problems of cystitis, bladder irritability, urgency and burning pains on passing water. Gonorrhoeal urethritis with white or yellow discharge. Prostatic enlargement with frequency.

Petzinger, Von Karl Johann Sigmund M.D. (1903–   )

The emminent contemporary German physician and homoeopath, who works mainly in Konigsberg. Chairman of the regional association of homoeopathic doctors of Nieder-Sachsen and since 1959, chairman of the self-dispensing homoeopathic doctors. He has been active in the International League as a teacher and organiser for many years.

Pharyngitis

Inflammation of the pharynx or soft tissues at the back of the throat and mouth, infective in origin. The condition may be either acute or chronic. Major symptoms are pain on swallowing, general soreness and redness of the area, with an infected yellowish-green mucous drip down into the back of the throat. The area feels hot and swollen.

REMEDIES

For acute cases consider *Aconitum, Belladonna, Phytolacca, Lachesis, Mercuris.*

In chronic cases consider *Baryta Carb, Arg. Nit., Sulphur.*

Phellandrium (Water drop wort)

The major spheres of action is on the breasts and respiratory tissues. Mainly a right-sided remedy. Indicated in chronic bronchitis and emphysema with chronic cough, shortness of breath and mucous production, often offensive and infected. Headache is common and often the head feels too large. Pain in the nipples between feeds when lactating is a characteristic of the remedy.

186

Phlebitis

Inflammation of the veins. The condition should always be medically treated because of the danger of embolus formation. The condition may be superficial from a local wound or bite or sometimes there is more generalised infection with involvement in the deep veins. The latter condition needs most careful attention and medical care. In some cases anticoagulant therapy is required. The condition of deep vein thrombosis may follow any operation or a severe prolonged physical illness with lengthy period of bed-rest. Symptoms are shooting pains in the area, tenderness, temperature with swelling, redness, tenderness or stiffness.

REMEDIES

Aconitum, Phosphorus, Hammamelis, Pulsatilla, Vipera, Lachesis.

Phosphoric Acid

First proved by Hahnemann. The remedy has marked action on the emotions, in particular symptoms of fatigue, exhaustion, drowsiness with depression. In contrast to *Opium,* the patient is more easily roused from the stupor-like state of apathy. Most of the excretory areas of the body are stimulated to drain and sicharge profusely so that there is a frequent passage of urine, discharge profusely so that there is a frequent passage of urine, value in the morose, grief-stricken, depressed when unable to rally or respond to reassurance and support (*Ignatia*).

Phosphorus (red phosphorus)

The remedy for sudden violent explosive outbursts of symptoms with burning pains everywhere. It is indicated in the tall, pale, fair or red-haired make-up, thin over-grown, and anaemic-looking. There are many chest symptoms, with cough, bronchitis, asthma, pneumonia, shortness of breath, blood in the sputum and flashes of burning pains in the stomach or intestine. Vomiting of mucous with watery diarrhoea is frequent. Typically they crave salt and ice-cold drinks.

Physostigma (Calabar Bean)

A remedy for spasm as in tetanus, spinal paralysis, poliomyelitis.

Vomiting, collapse, diarrhoea with a slow pulse and sweating. The pupil is pin-point as after a stroke. Spinal meningitis, palpitations. Useful in any chronic paralysing conditions as multiple schlerosis, motor neurome disease, hereditary ataxias with weakness, muscle wasting, loss of strength and power.

Phytolacca Decandra (Poke Root)

Tincture of the fresh root. Introduced to homoepathy by Hale and one of the best remedies for violent throat pains with soreness and swelling of the soft palate and pharanyx. Pain on swallowing and tonsillitis. Vomiting and diarrhoea, muscular cramps and rigidity, spasm or convulsion. The other main sphere of action is breast tissue where there is mastitis, cystic nodular breast problems, or a cracked nipple with soreness. The breasts are painful during the mentrual periods. Diptheria.

Pilocarpinum (Jaborandi)

An alkaloid which in homoeopathic form is indicated for night-sweats of the menopause or hyperthyroidism. Restlessness and irritability is common. There are many eyes problems where the remedy is recommended espcially eye fatigue, contracted pupil, lachrymation, short-sightedness.

Placebo

An inert, non-medicated substance, somtimes prescribed to observe the patient for a period without medication or to allow a prescribed remedy a greater period of prolonged action without interference but where it is felt that the patient nevertheless, during the interim waiting stage, needs psychological support. According to how the physician best judges the psychological needs and strengths of the patient, placebo may or may not be required.

Plantago (Plantain)

Tincture of the whole fresh plant. Introduced by Hale to Homoeopathy. It is a rather unusual remedy in that it is often used locally as the undiluted mother-tincture for toothache or painful haemorrhoids. Of especial value in abscess, dental neuralgia, trigeminal neuralgia, earache. It is also indicated where large amounts of urine are passed as in diabetes or enuresis. The anal area is indicated for severe pain from piles when inflammed. In general it is a left-sided remedy, all symptoms are worse for cold air, movement or excessive heat.

Platina (the metal Platinum)

Trituration of the element. Platina is a major remedy for hysteria and pride associated with depression, irritability and restlessness. There may be uncontrollable impulses to violence. Cramps, spasm, constipation and Pruritis vulvae are all common.

Plumbum Met (Lead)

Trituration of the element. An important remedy which has paralysis of certain groups of muscles, especially wrist-drop or weakness. Pains are severe, cramping or wandering with spasm of a colicy type. Constipation is absolute. Anal spasm. Gout. In general the patient is emaciated with loss of weight and exhaustion. There is a characteristic greyish-blue tinge to the skin. All symptoms are better from rest, warmth and firm local pressure. The typical lead colic is improved by warmth and doubling-up.

Pneumonia

Inflammation of the lung by either bacterial or viral infection. This is a serious condition with raised temperature — except in the elderly when it may be below normal. Cough sometimes of blood, shortness of breath, collapse. In all cases it is best treated by a physician or hospitalisation.
REMEDIES
Aconitum, Arsenicum, Lycopodium, Rhus Tox, Senega, Sulphur, Mercurius.

Podophyllum Pelatrum (Mandrake)

Tincture of the whole plant, first proved by Williamson. There are many bowel symptoms with griping, colicy abdominal pain, flatulence, weakness and diarrhoea. The stools are often watery or greenish and after their passage the patient feels faint. Rectal or

189

uterine prolapse, right-sided ovarian pain, vomiting of
pregnancy, haemorrhoids of pregnancy, are the other areas of
action.

Poisoning

Acute poisoning may be accidental or deliberately induced. The
commonest causes include infected or contaminated food as
mushroom poisoning, botulism from infected tinned food. Food
poisoning is usually salmonella. Carbon monoxide poisoning is
from fumes of exhaust motor gases in poorly ventilated areas.
Domestic gas before the age of natural gas was a common toxic
hazard and still is in some holiday centres with yearly fatalities.
Other forms of accidental poisoning are the ingestion of toxic
chemical substances used in the home — like weed killer or
caustic fluids — often stored in a lemonade bottle. Sedatives when
taken to excess may make the person confused or ill. Alcohol
poisoning can occur when a large quantity of strong alcohol is
rapidly consumed — either in error or otherwise. The acute cases
must be treated urgently, under medical care. Vomiting should be
induced by means of an emetic made from salt or mustard and
water. The patient must be removed from the toxic area and
treated for shock and kept warm.
REMEDIES
Arnica, Rescue Remedy, *Veratrum Alb, Aconitum.*

Chronic poisoning is often a problem of water or atmospheric
pollution and is increasingly an environmental hazard with lead,
carbon monoxide, at dangerous unacceptable levels and D.D.T.,
now globally distributed, as also radioactive cobalt and
strontium. The symptoms must be treated symptomatically by
the best and most appropriate remedy plus a combination of
political lobbying and avoidance of densely-populated toxic
urban areas whenever possible. Deliberate poisoning requires
forensic investigation as well as treatment if suspected.

Poliomyelitis (Infantile paralysis)

The acute viral illness with infiltration and inflammation of spinal
cord nerve roots leading to degeneration, paralysis and wasting of
certain muscle groups according to the degree of spinal root
infiltration. Depending upon the degree and severity of the
attack, the disease may affect facial, laryngeal, respiratory or limb

muscles with weakness, wasting or complete and permanent paralysis. The disease is infective and epidemic and preventable by the specific poliomyelitis vaccine. In recent years the disease has become rare in Europe although still endemic in other countries. Supportive homoeopathic remedies to the vaccine are *Gelsemium, Baryta Carb, Calc. Carb, Phosphorus, Arsenicum.* In all cases medical care is needed and hospitalisation when at all severe.

Pollen Sensitivity

Often an inherited problem with a family history of either hay-fever, asthma or eczema in one or both parents. The person affected is usually of sensitive nature, both psychologically and physiologically, and stress or anxiety heightens physical discomfort. The commonest problems are hay fever with conjuctivitis, itchy red eyes, itchy palate, sneezing, nasal congestion and tightness of the chest, with asthma. In some cases the condition becomes unrelated to pollen and more aggravated by dust, animal hair, or hot dry atmospheres and is present all the year around.

REMEDIES

Phosphorous, Kali Carb, or *Phleum pratens, House Dust, Mixed pollens, Dulcamara.*

Polyps

Enlargement and prolongation of the mucosa can occur in any part of the body where there is mucous membrane lining, including the large bowel, uterus, bladder and nasal mucosa. It is a frequent cause of bleeding and discharge with irritation and blockage in the area. The commonest area affected is the nose with swelling and oedema causing chronic nasal catarrh, mouth breathing, epistaxis (nose bleeding) and infective discharges. The polyps can frequently be seen on examination of the nostril.

REMEDIES

Thuja, Calc. Carb, Phosphorous, Sanguinaria, Kali Bic, Mercurius

Potency — homoeopathic

Refers to the strength or dilution of the remedy at each stage in its preparation. The higher the potency — for example a 200c or

10^{-400} dilution — the stronger the remedy. Each successive dilution, dynamised by the succussion process, enhances the strength, activity, depth and breadth of action of the remedy. Commonly the polycrests and the constitutional remedies are prescribed in the higher 200c potencies whilst a remedy used for a more local condition is given in the lower 6c dilution. Potency is the innate energy-factor used in the medicines — ultimately one of natures deepest and most effective catalyst-elements. A recent paper at the international congress of Vienna (1983) emphasised just these points. Professor Gutman and Resch demonstrated that homoeopathic potency is something quite different from the usual physical principles and models used, which are largely experimental, but do not occur as such in nature or man. Potency is not measurable by conventional instruments — designed to picks up energy charges of a different type. During trituration and succussion, a dynamic pattern is liberated which the solvent memorises, affecting molecular energy, giving a far greater speed of movement. This memory can be transmitted to glass as has been known to the homoeopathic pharmacist for many years and is present when water is used as a dilutant but enhanced by an alcohol mixture and succussion. They recommended the centisimal scale of dilution as being more effective than the decimal scale in the transmission of potency energy charges.

Pregnancy

There are no contradications to the use of homoeopathic remedies during pregnancy and it can be quite safely prescribed for morning sickness (*Cocculus, Nux Vom.*); miscarriage and threatened abortion of the 3rd month (*Sabina, Secale, Sepia, Caulophyllum*). Problems of the pregnant mother based on anxiety or fear, with tension, apprehension or intercurrent physical illness can also be treated without risk to mother or baby.

In the last four months of the pregnancy, *Caulophyllum* is given to stimulate healthy uterine tone and functioning and to make for a healthy smooth labour and delivery.

Prevention by homoeopathy

It is well-recognized that homoeopathy has an important role to play in prevention. A specific infectious disease, particularly prevalent at the time — in a child or near-neighbour may be best avoided for various reasons. Examples include *Belladonna* for measles prevention, *Pertussin* for whooping cough, *Merc. Cy.* for diptheria. The nosodes of mumps, german measles, glandular fever, chicken pox have a similar prophylactic action.

Primula Veris (cowslip)

Tincture of the fresh whole plant. The remedy is of value for problems of cerebral congestion, drowsiness or dullness with disorientation and confusion. Unsteadyness is common as from a threatened stroke or cerebral catastrophe when blood pressure suddenly becomes high and critical. The head is hot and there is headache or dizzyness with a sensation of fullness.

Principles of Homoeopathy

The science of homoeopathy is based on two major principles which are basic to the method:
1. A comparative study is made of the manifestations or external symptoms of the patient — the illness with those produced by the medical substances used in the treatment. This is called the Law of Similitudes when the two symptom patterns of patient and remedy are matched by the prescriber. For example coffee in its homoeopathic form of *Coffea* can be used in the treatment of some forms of insomnia, palpitations and agitation.
2. The therapeutic use of infinitesimal dosages produced by successive serial dilutions of the mother tincture, and therefore completely free from possible toxic side-effects of the medicaments used. Such substances are traditionally either vegetable, plant, animal or mineral in origin.

Prostate Problems

These include acute prostatis from bacterial or viral infection with pain and tenderness in the area, urinary irritation and discomfort. The commonest difficulty is benign enlargment of middle-age and elderly males with delay and difficulty in passing urine, frequency and a weak stream. Careful examination is necessary not to miss or mis-diagnose the rarer malignant growth of prostate which may for a time give similar symptoms.
REMEDIES
Solidago, Ferrum Pic, Chamomilla, Eupatorium Purp., Digitalis, Sabal Serrulata, Mercurius.

193

Proteus (Bach)

The bowel nosode for dark-haired, tense and irritable depressive temperaments prone to violent attacks of temper if crossed. Impulsive, sudden, with poor controls they are equally spasmodic in every part of them. There are for example sudden spasms in the blood supply to an area with angina, coronary thrombosis, intermittent claudication. Capillary spasm with 'dead' fingers. Equally there may be violent flashes of heat. Sour in temperament and in the stomach equally. Acidity, heartburn, hunger pains are typical. Constipation, anal itching and various contractions or contracures of tendons (*causticum*) especially the palms and little finger. Cramp, sudden and violent with associated irritability.

Provings

The experimental use of a homoeopathic potency by healthy volunteers who carefully record the results of taking different strengths of substance over a period of several weeks. Careful daily record is kept of all symptoms experienced including any particular sensitivity to the remedy — and more vigorous response. The totality is put together to complete the remedy-picture and indications for prescribing. The first early proving were carried out by Hahnemann, his family and colleagues, the remedy known to the provers. In recent years to avoid suggestion playing a role, the tendency has been to carry out double-blind proving trials where neither prover or physician in charge knows the identity of the remedy until after the experiment. With a totally new remedy of no known or published results, this is not necessary.

Pruritis

Itching of the skin, particularly common in the anal-genital area although it can occur in any part of the body. It is a distressing common problem and may at times be associated with haemorrhoids, varicose veins or sometimes infection of the area. Threadworm infection is common in adults as well as children, the itching characteristically occurring at night. Not uncommonly there has been a period of recent stress and strain causing pressure and emotional tension which is the major underlying factor.

REMEDIES

Caladium, Rhus Tox, Cina, Hammamelis, Rumex Crisp.

Psora

The most impòrtant of Hahnemann's three hereditary miasms, extensively developed in detail in his writings on chronic disease. It is considered that psora developed in a major way as a result of suppression of the 'itch' or scabies infection and according to Hahnemann this is the root of many of our present chronic disease problems. Major symptoms involve the skin with infection, cracking, also diarrhoea and chronic indigestion is common. Depression, apathy with exhaustion are other manifestations of psora.

Arsenicum, Aurum, Baryta Carb. Calc. Carb, Carbo Veg, Carb, Calc Carb, Carbo Veg, Causticum, Graphites, Hepar Sulph, Kali Carb, Mezereum, Petroleum, Phosphorus, Sulphur, Psorinum.

Psoriasis

The now common skin condition of unknown origin occuring in all age groups from childhood onwards. There are multiple areas of erruption with isolated thickened red patches which join-up, and may cover the entire body or an old area of injury. They have a silvery covering layer which tends to flake easily, causing itching and general discomfort. The lesions are disfiguring but heal without scar formation and usually completely. During the acute phase the face, scalp, trunk or limbs may be involved and cause psychological problems because of their unsightly nature. In some cases the nails, hands, joints or genital area is also involved. The results are generally encouraging with homoeopathic treatment.

REMEDIES

Mezereum, Natrum Mur, Psorinum, Graphites, Petroleum, Calcarea, Pulsatilla, Kali Arsen.

Psorinum (Scabies)

The nosode of psora, prepared from the infected scabies vesicle. It is one of the most valuable of all remedies. The main clinical indications are lack of concentration, depression with despair, an infected itch which discharges, or chronic skin conditions with offensive oozing and infection. There is general chillyness, the skin dirty-looking, the sweat offensive as the diarrhoea. Canine hunger, which is insatiable is typical and often diagnostic plus weakness and shortness of breath on the least exertion.

Ptelea Trifolata (Water Ash)

A useful remedy for chronic liver problems where there is tenderness and enlargement. Hepatitis. The liver area feels painful — like a dragging weight, pulling down, the whole of the upper right upper abdominal region uncomfortable and worse for lying on the right side. Chronic indigestion and rheumatic problems, usually right-sided (*Lycopodium*).

Puberty

The onset of breast changes and the menstrual cycle in the girl, secondary sexual changes — pubic hair and emissions in the boy as a preparation for reproduction and adult life. It is a time of major hormonal and psychological adjustment. The age of onset is getting younger with successive generations as general health and nutrition of the population improves. The average age of menstrual onset is now from 12–14 years with a wide range of difference on either side of this figure. When early periods are either delayed or variable and irregular, *Pulsatilla 6* is often of help. Where the child is late in developing generally and sexual development is obviously retarded in an overall way, consider *Calc. Carb* or *Silicea*.

Pulsatilla Nigrans (Anemone Pratensis)

Tincture of the fresh flowering plant. The remedy is indicated whenever there is great change and variability of mood or symptoms, and is especially helpful in the female although not solely. In general the temperament is passive, compliant, frequently tearful but at the same time quickly changing to one of stubborness and anger before returning to becoming the peacemaker and too easy-going. There are many chronic digestive catarrhal problems with exhaustion, chillyness and discomfort on the warmest day — either from feeling cold or intolerance of heat. Profuse weeping is a common feature. Because of considerable congestion and a tendency to fluid-retention, thirst is usually completely lacking. Fats are as disagreeable to *Pulsatilla* as heat and both cause suffering and discomfort.

Quin, Harvey Foster, M.D. (1799-1878)

The emminent homoeopath who first introduced homoeopathy to this country. He was particularly impressed by the approach at an early age, soon after qualifying and especially by the results of homoepathy in the Paris cholera epidemic of 1831. He had enormous influence on our earliest English homeopaths and formed the first English Homoeopathic Society in 1837. He was founder-president of the British Homoepathic Society in 1844. The London Homoeopathic Hospital was also formed under his influence in 1844 where he began teaching and held comprehensive courses of clinical tuition. His major literary contribution was *Materia Medica Pura* in 1838.

Quinsy

The condition of peritonsillar abscess, usually on one side only, with a high temperature, severe pain, toxicity and a choking sensation. The whole tonsil area is severely inflammed and enlarged, the child ill, with vomiting and sometimes collapse from fever.

REMEDIES

Aconitum, Baryta Carb, Silicea, Sulphur, Merc. Sol., Hepar Sulph.
Fortunately the condition has now become rare. In severe cases given Penicillin because of the virulence of the infection or where there is a danger of general toxicity overwhelming the vital response.

199

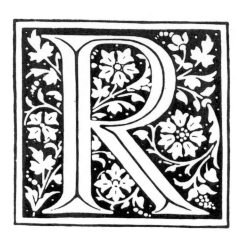

Rademacher, Johann Gottfried (1772–1850) M.D.

The early medical practitioner, working mainly from Goch in North-Western Germany during the first half of the 19th century. He was a keen observer and disciple and admirer of Paracelsus. In 1841 he published his major work in German — *Universal and Organ Remedies* in two volumes, 800 pages each. Here he developed his principle theory of organ correspondences, or remedies having special affinity for certain parts of the body. He was important because his ideas affected medical thinking for several generations and he firmly laid the emphasis of disease on the organ involved and the pathology of disease, also in chronic illness. To this extent he was in opposition to Hahnemann's ideas of more overall symptoms, including the mentals and modalities being of key importance for prescribing. Rademacher was supported by both Hughes, Burnett and others. See for example Burnetts monographs on 'Diseases of the Liver and Spleen.'

Raeside, John Robertson, M.D. (1926–1971)

One of the victims of the tragic Trident air disaster of 1971 which took so many young and promising homoeopaths, travelling together to the Brussels International Congress of that year. Raeside especially was pre-emminent in his group. Born in Glasgow and educated in that city, he had a natural sensitivity towards the philosophy of Steiner which he supported all his life. Formerly assistant to Dr. Blackie, he played an important role in the field of new remedy provings and gave a revival of interest to a difficult area with a series of well-presented and scientific papers over several years. He was the spearhead of research at the faculty up to the time of his death.

Ranunculus Bulb (Buttercup)

Essentially a remedy for muscular rheumatism with stiching tearing pains of chest and spine. The symptoms are aggravated by fear (*Aconitum*). The patient feels weak and faint. Pleurisy with burning pains on breathing-in, all symptoms generally aggravated by damp or cold air. The same burning pains may involve the bladder or stomach. Chronic alcoholism with hiccough, shingles, skin irritation with redness, vesicle formation, itchy and irritable.

Raphanus Sativus (the Black Radish)

Flatulence with a sensation of a bubble of air in the stomach that cannot be released. (*Kali Carb.*) It is specially valuable in post operative paralysis or atony of the alimentary tract.

Ratanhia (Krameria)

Tincture of the root. The remedy acts on the large bowel with constipation of hard, dry painful stools causes much straining and pressure leading to severe haemorrhoids. The piles are painful and burning after a motion. There are two bizarre but characteristic diagnostic symptoms — the rectum often feels like splinters of glass (*Thuja*), and the back teeth seem to have a sensation of cold water running through them.

Rau, Charles Gottlieb. M.D. (1820–1836)

The early 19th century German homoeopathic physician.
His major works include:
1871 *Elements of Psychology*
1868 *Subjective and Objective symptoms*
1868 *Special Pathological and diagnosis*
1870 *Mental symptoms*
1870–75 *The annual record of homoeopathic literature*
1884 *A memorial of Constantine Hering*

1889 *Psychology as a natural science.*
Also co-editor of Hering's *Guiding Symptoms*, he wrote some of the earliest and most important volumes on psychology emphasising the importance of the mentals for prescribing.

Rauwolfia (Apocyanea)

A recently proved remedy having a valuable role to play in irritable depression and raised blood pressure with palpitations, headache and shortness of breath.

Raynaud's Disease

Arterial spasm from hypersensitivity of the circulatory system usually due to cold. It occurs at any age, affecting particularly the hands, with the finger tips becoming lifeless and white. At other times the fingers are red, mauve, tingling and itching. The problem can occur in young men associated with excessive cigarette smoking. Often there is a family disposition going back over several generations. Rarely it can lead to gangrene and loss of limb in the particularly severe form of the disease.
REMEDIES
Silicea, Pulsatilla, Agaricus, Nux Vom, Secale.

Reactions to Homoeopathy

Deficient reactions when there is no lasting response to the well-prescribed remedy may occur in the elderly with low vital energy levels. It sometimes occurs after a long taxing illness which has depleted energy reserves from chronic illness or mechanical organic obstructions, strictly surgical rather than a homoeopathic conditions. For failure to respond — other than in obstructive problems, Boenninghausen recommended the following *Carbo Veg. Laurocerasus, Opium, Sulphur, Thuja,* prescribed according to the overall picture as is basic to the method. A nosode should also be considered as *Medorrhinum, Psorinum, Tub. Bov, Syphilinum.* Excessive reactions need a different approach. A more severe aggravation sometimes occurs when steriods have occured — causing 'bounce-back', symptoms having been held artificially, just under the surface until the homoeopathic remedy comes into effect to release them and a 'Jack in the box' reaction occurs. Similarly with prolonged and unsatisfactory allopathic treatment, a more severe aggravation may occur. Such excessive reactions are nearly always unavoidable and do not reflect wrong or inaccurate prescribing but rather the start of a homoeopathic reaction after years of suppression in some cases. Boenninghausen recommended for such severe reactions, *Asafoetida, Chamomilla, Coffea, China, Ignatia, Nux Vom, Sulphur, Teucrium, Valerium.* In all cases the most appropriate remedy must be chosen to fit the patient's overall symptom-picture.

Reappearance of earlier Symptoms

During the course of homoeopathic treatment, it is quite common and 'normal' for earlier suppressed and usually inadequately treated or suppressed illness — sometimes from years previously, to re-emerge as isolated symptoms from the past. Only rarely does it reappear as a more severe illness — usually transient and fragmentary in passage. Nevertheless such symptoms are important and significant revealing that they have been underlying factors in the more recent illness that has brought the patient to treatment. Once they have emerged and been treated by the appropriate homoeopathic prescription they do not recur. Examples are the recurrance of an old and forgotten gonorrhoeal infection which recurs as a discharge with no recent cause for it. Others seen are a return of hay-fever or transient asthma. The patient usually makes better progress once these underlying suppressed factors have come out and been dealt with.

Recovery by the Homoeopathic Method

Both patient and physician must fully realise that the response to homoeopathy follows a clear-cut order and natural law of response. In all cases, whatever the problem or remedy prescribed, recovery always proceeds from the centre outwards — a cardiac symptom like angina recovers before a joint or skin disability. It also occurs from above downwards — the scalp and face clear in chronic psoriasis or eczema before the trunk or limbs. Symptoms disappear in reverse order of appearance and the most recent symptoms are cured first — those of longest duration last of all. It is not uncommon in heart disease for the patient to complain that they are no better. On examination the palpitations breathlessness and angina pain have quite gone but the patient now has rheumatic pains. This means that the process of homoeopathic cure has begun exactly according to expectation. But how common for the patient to quickly forget earlier problems and to complain of being worse rather than better, with yet another prescription given for a condition that has really evolved and improved.

Rectal Prolapse

Protusion of rectal musosa from lack of tone or muscular weakness as may follow a debilitating illness, loss of weight, severe strain, surgery in the pelvic area, childbirth, chronic severe constipation.
REMEDIES
Podophyllum, Arg. Nit, Carb. Sulphur, Fluor. Ac., Hydrastis, Phosphorus, Syphilinum.

Renal Colic

The condition of severe abdominal pain due to the passage of a renal calculus along the ureter. The pain is cramping and unbearable causing shock, weakness and collapse. In general the condition is eased by doubling-up and local heat.
REMEDIES
Mag. Phos, Nux. Vom, Senec., Dioscorea, Berberis, Urtica.

Repertory

The reference book of all homoeopathic physicians containing the totality of all the recorded proving symptoms classified and related to the appropriate remedy and according to general and particular symptoms and their modalities. A patient is repertorised when the total symptom-picture is matched against the repertory listing in order to decide which remedy fits the majority of the symptoms. The most extensive and best known repertories are those of Kent — which is widely used, and that of Boenninghausen. In recent months the repertory has been computer-programmed for apparent speed and convenience.

Repetition of the Remedy

It is a fundamental rule of homoeopathic practise not to repeat the prescribed remedy as long as the patient is improving. When prescribing for more local conditions in low 6c or 3X potencies — these should be stopped as soon as the condition has completely cleared. They need not be further repeated unless there is a recurrence when a different potency or remedy is required.

Resonance

The homoeopathic concept of the affinity of a specific remedy for the particular patient and his unique patterns of symptoms and needs at a given time. When the remedy is 'right' and matches the patient, it is in resonance and a vital reaction occurs, manifested by external changes in the symptom-pattern and an increase in available energy and well-being. At deeper levels, there also arises a change in the internal dynamics with a freeing of fixed areas of stress or non-functioning, beginning with the most recent, uppermost layers of rigidity and statis. This freeing will always occur provided that the problem is not one of a severe immovable mechanical nature or blockage that requires surgery — when homoeopathy is not indicated or advised.

Rest — importance of

During the course of homoeopathic treatment, regular habits are recommended with a rhythmic life and routine as much as possible. Avoidance of excesses, including tea, coffee, tobacco and highly spiced foods is advisable and attention to the quality and amount of food taken. This is to encourage conservation of vital energy and reserves made more available to the vital curative response.

Restlessness

Due to organic disease and damage to the central nervous system, or temperamental factors and accumulation of nervous energy from worry and stress that cannot be dispersed. Symptoms include tension, restlessness, agitation, insomnia and anxiety.
REMEDIES
Arsenicum, Nux Vom, Medorrhinum, Zinc. Met.

208

Retarded Milestones

The causes are variable and careful attention must be given to the history and any investigations felt to be in the patient's best interests. Common problems include Subnormality, Down's Syndrome (Mongolism), Vitamin or hormonal deficiency diseases; Diet and nutritional factors; familiar causes; mental illness, infection and chronic disease.

REMEDIES

Calc. Carb., Silicea, Sulphur, Baryta Carb, Tub. Bov, Medorrhinum.

Retention of Urine

The inability to pass urine, usually due to spasms of the sphincter or a fibrous stricture from earlier disease. In some common cases the cause is trauma of the bladder expulsive muscles after surgery in the area with temporarily paralysis. Other causes may be blockage from a bladder calculus or prostatic disease.

REMEDIES

Causticum, China, Thuja, Sabal Serrulata, Opium, Cantharis.

Rheumatic Fever

The acute generalised allergic condition of young people due to haemolytic streptococcal infection of the throat. The throat is severely infected, the joints inflamed with redness and swelling with frequent involvement of the pericardium leading to pericarditis and inflammation of the heart valves, especially the mitral valve. If scarring occurs there may be mitral stenosis and narrowing in adult years unless the condition is thoroughly treated at the time.

REMEDIES

A course of penicillin is essential to avoid the risks of cardiac complications. All cases must be under the care of an experienced physician. Recommended homoeopathic remedies include *Aconitum, Bryonia, Mercurius, Rhus Tox, China, Sulphur, Pulsatilla, Crataegus.*

Rheumatism

This is usually muscular in origin from changes in the muscles and tendons acting like a barometer — expanding and contracting with atmospheric pressure and aggravated by damp or cold. Such changes pull on tiny nerve fibres of the tendon and muscle sheath causing pain. When it occurs in the low back area it produces acute lumbago. Often chronic because of our damp climate and island conditions, it is more of a nuisance than anything else. Stress of any kind always aggravates the condition, as does strain and fatigue.

REMEDIES
Rhus Tox, Bryonia, Dulcamara, Causticum, Medorrhinum.

Rheumatoid Arthritis

The common acute inflammatory joint condition of unknown origin. It is probably an allergic reaction but this is still unproven. The condition is commoner in females of the 20-40 year age group than in the male. There is no cardiac involvement. Swelling, pain, stiffness with raised temperature, loss of use due to pain with muscle wasting and distortion of joints can occur. Depression of mood is frequent. The condition may resolve completely or become chronic with joints and movement rigid and fixed from fibrosis.

REMEDIES
Apis, Natrum Mur, Medorrhinum, Belladonna, Aconitum, Causticum. The constitutional prescription.

Rhinitis

Inflammation of nasal mucosa with thickening and congestion leading to catarrhal discharge, varying with the type and degree of infection.

REMEDIES
Pulsatilla, Calcarea, Kali Carb. Sulphur.

Rhododendron (Rhododendron Chrysanthum)

Mainly a remedy for rheumatic problems with pain and spasm of fibrous and muscular tissue and great sensitivity to changes of climate. All symptoms are aggravated by an impending electric or thunder storm and better after the storm has passed. Damp also aggravates as does prolonged sitting or inactivity. Generally better for movement and exercise. The testicle may be involved with epidymitis.

Rhus Tox (American Poison Ivy)

One of the most useful of all homoeopathic remedies. The mood is one of restlessness irritability and anxiety. It acts on skin, muscle and fibrous tissue around the joints. Of particular value in rheumatic conditions where there is pain, stiffness and incapacity. All symptoms are worse from immobility of any type — sitting or sleeping. The skin is red, irritated, swollen with vesicle formation. Shingles. Cold and damp aggravate the rheumatic pains and stiffness but they are relieved by heat and movement.

Right-sided Homoeopathic Remedies

Certain remedies have a predisposition for one side of the body and act strongly on problems in these areas. The major right-acting remedies are *Lycopodium, Colocynth, Diosorea, Napthalinum, Indigo, Mag. Phos., Palladium, Tellurium.*

Rosa Canina (Dog Rose)

Tincture of ripe hips. Proved by Compton-Burnett. A remedy for chronic bladder and prostrate problems with difficulty and slowness in passing urine.

Rosemarinus Officinalis (Rosemary)

Tincture of the whole plant. One of our most ancient remedies. The main indications are alopocia, poor concentration and memory (*Lycopodium*).

Ross, Andrew Christie Gordon, M.D. (1904-1932)

Educated in Glasgow, Ross studied medicine at St. Andrews, working and practising in Glagow for most of his life. He worked as an enthusiastic homoeopath, following the traditions of his older brother Douglas. A keen golfer, he was also an author and playwrite. Especially he was prolific in his homoeopathic articles with over 200 to his credit in various journals. His major written

211

contributions are *Homoeopathy – an introductory study; Arnica, the amazing healer; Homoeopathic Green Medicine.*

Ross, Thomas Douglas, M.D. (1902-1964)

The eminent Scottish homoeopath, educated at Glasgow University. Superintendent and later consultant to the Glasgow Homoeopathic Hospital, he was president of the faculty from 1962-64. A keen golfer, musician and prolific writer, he had a keen appreciation of the uniqueness of the individual which was one of the major reasons for his very high regard, standards and eminence as a physician and prescriber.

Royal, George, M.D. (1853–   )

The American homoeopath. President of homoeopathic materia medica and therapeutics in the state university of Iowa for 30 years. Also president and chairman of the Council of Medical Education of the American Institute of Homoeopathy. Member of the Hahnemann Medical Association of Iowa and honourary member of the British Homoeopathic Medical Society.
His major writings include:
A textbook of the homoeopathic theory and practise of medicine.

Royal London Homoeopathic Hospital

Founded by Quin in 1844. Initially in Golden Square, it played an important role in its early days during the Cholera epidemic of 1854 when homoeopathic treatments were so successful that the mortality rate for the disease was only 16% compared with 52% in all other hospitals. There was considerable hostility to homoeopathy at the time and Quin was instrumental in ensuring tht these figures were not suppressed and also that there was security of practice for the homoeopathic physicians of his time when attempts were made to outlaw them. The hospital still plays a major role with both in-patient and out-patient clinical work. There is an attached surgical unit with a new operating theatre due to be opened in 1983. Homoeopathic doctors are assured a thorough training over the three year period of qualification and regular post-graduate meetings and lectures are held. The faculty of the hospital is responsible for the teaching programme and the bi-annual membership examination. The high standard of teaching and clinical training ensures wide interest, with doctors coming from many countries. At present, the faculty probably offers the best homoeopathic training in the world.

Royal Patronage

Homoeopathy has been very fortunate to have considerable royal support over many years. H.M. Queen Elizabeth is patron of the Royal London Homoeopathic Hospital, The Queen Mother, patron of the British Homoeopathic Association. There has been a homoeopathic physician appointed to the royal household since Sir John Weir, followed by Dr. Blackie and recently Dr. Elliott.

Ruddock, Edwin Harris, M.D. (1822-1865)

The eminent English homoeopathic practitioner. Trained at Guys and Barts who qualified from Edinburgh in 1865. Editor of the Homoeopathic World.
His major writings include:
A Ladies manual of home treatment,
Stepping stones to homoeopathy and health.
Homoeopathic Vade-Mecum — (his most important work, later revised by Wheeler and Clarke).
Consumption and tuberculous of the Lungs.
Diseases of Infants and Children
Pocket manual of homoeopathic vetinary medicine.

Rumex Crisp (Yellow Dock)

Titration of the whole flowering plant. Indicated for catarrh — thick, mucous-laden and abundent, mainly from the nasal and respiratory mucosa and severely congested. Morning diarrhoea is a feature (*Sulph.*). Pruritis improved by heat and worse for cold. All symptoms are generally better for heat and aggravated by cold or the least draught.

Ruta Grav. (Rue)

Titration of the leaves and young flowering buds. A remedy for fibrous tissues and tendons, in particular where there has been recent strain. Tearing, burning pains are common with a sensation of bruising (*Arnica*). There is nodular thickening in the tendons and peri-osteal membrane. Contractures of tendons may occur in chronic rheumatic illness, the hand drawn up or permanently fixed in a claw-shape or the foot permanently flexed and unusable. Particularly the flexor tendons are affected by the contractures (*Causticum*). It is also an important eye remedy for strain, and fatigue with pain or blurring of vision. The remedy has a role in chronic knee and hip problems. All symptoms are worse for cold, damp weather conditions or strain but often relieved by warm rain.

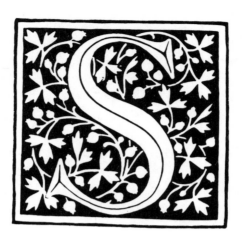

Sabadilla (Veratrum Sabadilla)

Tincture of the pulverised seeds and capsule. Mainly a left-sided remedy, for chronic catarrhal throat conditions, pains travelling to the right side of the throat or body. (*Lachesis, Lycopodium*). Mucous membrane is inflammed, particularly of the mouth, throat and palate, the upper respiratory tract frequently involved. Hay fever with sneezing is frequent also associated conjunctivitis. Tape worm infection. Anxiety of a hysterical nature with disturbance of body image. There is a general chillyness, all symptoms better for warmth and aggravated by the smell of flowers or fruit.

Sabal Serrulata (The Sabal palm)

Tincture of the fruit. A specific prostate remedy for congestion and pain with urinary discomfort. Major symptoms are a slow, weak stream with hesitancy or complete blockage of flow and retention. Cystitis and pain during the sexual act are a further indication. *Sabal* is often used as the mother tincture or in very low potencies for prostatic infection or enlargement.

Sabina (Savine)

A pelvic remedy where there is inflammation and bleeding from either rectal or anal regions or uterus and bladder. The area affected is painful and swollen with throbbing burning pain

217

leading to cystitis, urgency and stangury. Exhaustion is common. The periods are disturbed, heavy, prolonged with clots and sudden shooting or bearing-down pains. (cp. *Sepia*). Indicated for threatened abortion of the third month. The remedy also has varicose veins and anal warts.

Salicylic Acid

For problems of tinnitus with vertigo, the ear-noises like loud bells or high-pitched, with dizzyness, nausea. The face is hot and red. Meniere's Disease.

Salivary glands — problems of

Cysts may appear when a duct becomes blocked, especially the parotid gland. These are often firm, pea-sized, more of a nuisance and unsightly than a risk to health. In some cases they enlarge and then disappear, only to recur again at a later date for no obvious reason.
REMEDIES
Parotidinum, Silicea, Baryta Carb, Calc. Carb.

The salivary glands may become infected locally as with mumps or bacterial infection and cause abcess with pain and swelling.
REMEDIES
Merc. Sol, Pyrogenium, Belladonna.

Sometimes in the elderly the flow of saliva is excessive leading to dribbling in an otherwise health person.
REMEDIES
Merc Sol 6.

When there is a complete absence of flow of saliva, the mouth, tongue and palate dry, consider *Nux Moschata, Bryonia, Lycopodium.*

Salpingitis

Inflammation of the fallopian tubes — either acute or chronic. The commonest causes are bacterial or viral infection although chronic causes include tuberculosis. The cause needs careful diagnosis and treatment to avoid damage, scarring and blockage because of the dangers of sterility.

For acute cases *Arsenicum, Belladonna, Lachesis, Aconitum, Mercurius.*

For chronic cases consider *Medorrhinum, Sulphur, Tub. Bov, Graphites, Thiosinaminum.*

Salvia (Sage)

Tincture of the fresh leaves and flowers. Indicated for chronic throat problems with dry irritating cough and chronic gum infections with pus.

Sambucus Niger (Elder)

A remedy for oppressive states of fear and anxiety often associated with a high-pitched laryngitis and hoarseness.

Sanguinaria Canadensis (Blood Root)

A right-sided remedy for chronic nasal and throat conditions with catarrh, bronchitis, hay fever, bronchitis and winter colds. There is general weakness and exhaustion with tendency to migraine and vomiting. Circulatory problems with hot flushes and palpitations are common.

Santoninum (Santonin)

A remedy for worm parasitic infection especially thread-worms, with the typical irritation of the anal area and itchy nose. Stabismus or squinting associated with worms. Cataract. Vomiting and diarrhoea. There is a chronic cystitis with burning pains, difficulty in passing water, frequency. Nocturnal enuresis.

Sarsaparilla (Smilax)

A bladder remedy for chronic states of weakness and exhaustion. An odd symptom is the inability to pass water when standing, but freely when sitting. Bladder stones, the urine thick with sandy deposits. Enuresis, nocturia, gout, chronic constipation may also be present.

Scarlet Fever

The acute infection of childhood. The characteristic bright-red rash occurs first on covered areas of the body before involving the face and body totally. Sore throat with a raised temperature is usual and in severe cases the kidney is involved. The disease is highly infectious. In recent years the disease has fortunately followed a more benign course and seen less frequently than in earlier years when mortality was high in epidemics. Sporadic cases of the severe form occur but in general they are rare, although they occasionally give all the major complications. Medical care is essential.

REMEDIES

Belladonna 6 for prevention. For established cases consider *Aconitum, Belladonna* — the most important remedy, *Merc. Sol., Bryonia, Rhus Tox, Lachesis, Sulphur, Arsenicum.*

Schizophrenia

The acute psychotic mental illness, marked by withdrawal, isolation and a break from reality. Delusional thinking with hallucinations and ideas of reference are characteristic. It occurs in young people especially when the background is unstable, or there is an intolerable pressure-situation — for example a university student on a maintenance-grant, pressured by work, tutor and family. There may be a suicidal risk in some cases.

REMEDIES

Nat. Mur, Aurum Met, Medorrhinum, Stramonium, Sulphur, Arg. Nit.

Schmidt, Pierre, M.D. (1894–   )

The eminent contemporary homoeopath and teacher. Graduate of Geneva, he saw as a young man his father's chronic enteritis treated effectively by homoeopathy when all else had failed. Years later, in 1918, he experienced the value of the 200 C. potency of influenzinum nosodum during the 'flu epidemic. He has been one of the major forces of homoeopathic principles in both France and Switzerland. Formerly assistant at the Royal London Homoeopathic Hospital, he knew and worked with Clarke and Weir. Later he went to Philadelphia and met Kent and his principles of the single remedy and high potency prescribing.

Founder of the Hahnemannian group in Lyon, he has worked mainly in research and post-graduate studies. Founder-member of the International league and honourary president, Schmidt has translated into French some of Hahnemann's major works. These include his *Materia Medica, Chronic Diseases* and the sixth edition of the *Organon*. He is known for his many papers on philosophy, materia medica and clinical cases throughout a distinguished career. In 1955 at the 200th centenary celebrations of Hahnemann's birth, he gave a lecture on The Legacy of Hahnemann. He is now retired and lives in Nancy (France). He is still regarded as the doyen of Swiss homoeopathy. In 1960 he reported that a veterinary pupil of his had outstanding results in Foot and Mouth disease using the fresh Nosode prepared yearly in the 30, 200 and 1M potency with *Nitric Acid 6*.
Author of *Defective Illness (1980)*.

Schuessler, Willhelm Heinrich, M.D. (1898-1921)

The eminent 19th C. homoeopathic physician. Born in Germany, he studied medicine in both Berlin and Paris. He was founder of the Biochemic system, using 12 basic salts to restore cellular vitality and balance. It is largely an off-shoot of homoeopathy because it attempts to concentrate on cellular activity only and ignores the mentals and overall features and symptoms. Classical theory regards such cellular inbalance as a largely secondary phenomena. His *Twelve Tissue Remedies* was published in 1880.

Schultz Law

Developed by the experimental physiologists Arndt and Shultz. Working with minute plants and yeasts they found that small stimuli enhances growth, medium stimuli impedes it and strong stimuli destroys activity. The effect of *Arsenicum* on yeast cells has confirmed this with a weak solution stimulating cellular growth and a strong solution destroying growth and life. We can equate the homoeopathic potency with a weak stimulating solution to vital energy and responses and a strong solution with the suppressant drugs — destroying life and activity in the area. This is clearly seen after massive doses of an antibiotic when the patient may take days or even weeks to recover from it in terms of normal physiological functioning.

Sciatica

Pain due to irritation of the sciatic nerve. There is a dull ache in the buttock along the root of the nerve — often referred down the back or side of the thigh and lower limb to the ankle. Causes are variable and include herniation of an intervertebral disc with severe paralysing symptoms, due to vertebral displacement and requiring osteopathic re-alignment. At other times, disease of the spine or pelvis may irritate the spinal sciatic nerve roots and cause the symptom.

REMEDIES

Rhus Tox, Aconitum, Arsenicum, Nux. Vom, Colocynth, Chamomilla, Tellurium, Mag. Phos, Bryonia, Causticum, Plumbum.

Scientific Principles of Homoeopathy

Homoeopathy is prescribed by matching the proving, toxicology and clinical pictures of the remedy to the clinical symptomatology and overall picture of the patient. The assumption by the physician is that when the remedy-picture matches the patient, there will be a consistent vital reaction in terms of clinical change and symptoms according to established laws of homoeopathic response. This is the essence of homoeopathy and it meets all the criteria of the scientific method by testing a hypothesis and predicting an outcome in a consistent method of approach.

In the science of aerodynamics, the computer is used extensively. With careful input of data, mathematically sound, it is possible to exactly predict the flight pathway of the next generation of aerobus — their speed, efficiency, fuel-consumption and cost-efficiency.Models can be developed from the computer data to exactly simulate flight pathways and to predict and correct faults which are likely to develop — at a stage where the plane has barely left the drawing board.

However if you feed into the computer, similar data for the weight, size, wing-span and frequency of wing-movement for the bumble-bee, the computer comes up with the conclusion that it cannot fly. The fault is not in the computer, it lies in the particular form of data supplied with its inherent limits and boundaries and when these are exceeded it gives a wrong or negative response — because the computer is only designed to evaluate and process the particular type of data which is normally fed into it. This is the same problem with the common criticism of homoeopathy — that it does not work because it does not and cannot conform to the particular criteria of the double-blind method. Like the computer, it is designed solely to evaluate its own particular brand of data. Again the fault is not that of homoeopathy or that it is inconsistent, invalid or unscientific, but lies with the method of evaluation and apprasial of the experimental model. Concepts of double-blind and cross-over experiments are recent innovations and lead to poor results because it is impossible to exactly match one human or group of humans with another similar group. They just don't exist and approximately is not good enough in this area of prediction and response.

These are however purely points of technique and do not relate to a basic scientific method of approach. Much of the recent talk of the value of statistics is in fact very suspect when considering scientific method because it can be endlessly manipulated to fit the results and to either validate or invalidate them. They are largely irrelevent to sound scientific methods which in homoeopathy are based on clinical studies and clinical results. The 'scientifics' are doubly blind themselves — because all too often they fail to see the limitations and bias of their own models and to appreciate the true merits of alternative methods like homoeopathy which though clinically sound, fail to fit into their own particular brand of data-evaluation and logic.

The major area of criticism of homoeopathy has not been so much about its method or principles but concerns the use of infinitely small dilutions — beyond the molecular or material limit. The electron-microscope has in recent years considerably extended our scope and knowledge of cellular life functioning and structure to the extent that most of our physiology and neuro-physics is now being re-written and re-thought.

In war, we now use the single Exocet missile — on dot on a radar screen, fired from something approaching thirty miles away at a blob on a similar radar screen — yet capable of destroying a battle-ship which is invisible to the naked eye. It is only deviated from its target and inevitable 'hit' by a smoke-screen of similar radar micro heat-blobs. Likewise the sub-microscope virus can create devastation in the human organism, once it has gained entry into the physiological soil with vitality and resistance minimal.

Opium has been used in medicine for thousands of years very

effectively, and no one has really doubted its importance or validity. Yet is is only in very recent years that some understanding has emerged as to its mode of action by secreting minute opium-like endorphins at nerve endings within the central nervous system. In a similar way we are only now beginning to understand how Homoeopathy works, although its action is beyond doubt. The true action of Aspirin as a pain-killer is still not fully understood physiologically — but we know that it can be an effective pain-killer, even if not homoeopathic in principle and a suppressant.

The importance of essential trace elements as copper, manganese, cobalt, present in minute amounts, has only recently been more fully appreciated and made measurable as new techniques develop — often from such varied fields as space-technology and satellite studies. Similarly vitamins are required in minute quantities to ensure health.

As we enter into the age of nuclear medicine from nuclear war, it is likely that the true significance of the infinitesimal and the single dosage in potency will be more widely appreciated. Homoeopathy by imprinting its blue-print on the dilution and succession, energises and organises the solution. But measureable proof of this is still being researched and as throughout the whole of medicine scientific proof of a remedy and method lags behind every-day clinical evidence of its efficiency and value for the patient.

We are still awaiting further developments in nuclear medicine to give us the measuring instrument to accurately differentiate and measure our potencies, to record their unique energy patterns and levels of specificity. There have already been several experiments in the past which have shown the stimulant effect of potencies of up to 10^{-17} on algae growth and isolated muscles of the frog's heart. The 6c potency of *Phosphorus* 10^{-12}, has been shown to measurably regenerate rat liver cells, poisoned with Carbon Tetrachloride. But homoeopathy is not based or built-up on animal experiments and we await an outcome of confirmation at a more human level.

Such delay in no way detracts from the homoeopathic method or the scientific principles of the approach. The homoeopath is daily extending his patients by the potencies, freeing bound-up static energy to cure disease and at the same time freeing the patient for a fuller, more meaningful life. In many ways it is not up to homoeopathy to catch up with science but for science to catch up with homoeopathy.

Sea Sickness

The common problem of motion sickness at sea — worse for inclement weather, another person being ill which acts as a psychological stimulus to vomiting, or the smell of diesel oil.

REMEDIES

Arg nit., Arnica, Cocculus, Nux Vom, Petroleum, Berberis. Tabacum.

Seasonal Factors in homoeopathic prescribing

Some remedies have an optimum sphere or power of action at certain times of the year. This is not easily explainable but may in certain instances bear a relationship to the time at which the plant flowers are picked for preparation of the tincture — its intrinsic energy being at peak at this time. *Pulsatilla* is a mainly a spring remedy, *Sabadilla* works best in late spring and early summer. *Sulphur* acts best with the new moon, *M.A.P.* is primarily a late summer and early autumn remedy.

Secale Cornutum (Rye Ergot)

A circulatory remedy for burning pains, the area affected becoming bluish, numb and irritated with tingling — like 'pins and needles'. The toes and fingers may become black and gangrenous. Ulceration may occur. All symptoms are worse from heat and better for cold air (in contrast to *Sulphur*). Spasms and convulsions are characteristic with a tendency to bleeding. Dryness of the skin and mucous membrane with catarrh. Paralysis, numbness, sterility, recurrent miscarriage are the other features.

Selenium (Red Selenium)

Indicated for general weakness and exhaustion with weight loss, emaciation and paralysis. Depression, alopoecia, alcoholism, impotency. A tendency to bladder weakness with leaking on walking or movement (*Causticum*). Chronic laryngitis.

225

Senecio Aureus (Golden Ragwort)

Mainly a remedy for young women with menstrual problems. The periods are either suppressed or absent or there is excessive colicy pain on the first day. The cause of the missed periods can be chill, excessive travelling — overland or by plane in air-hostesses. Tuberculosis, chronic catarrh, hemorrhagic tendencies with violent nose bleeds, cystitis, renal failure. There is a typical dry 'rattling' cough at night.

Sepia Officinalis (Ink of the Cuttlefish)

One of Hahnemann's major anti-psoric remedies and known since antiquity as a medicine for female problems. It is primarly for the tall, thin, rather sallow woman, often strangely indifferent to those around her — as can occur quite commonly in puerperal depression. They are nervous, moody, irritable and feel worn-out — often totally lacking in joy or any form of response. At the end of the day the woman feels quite exhausted. There is frequently a saddle-shaped brown mark across the bridge of the nose. They feel old, dragged-down by pain, fatigue and chronic back-ache. Pelvic pain with uterine prolapse is common — the pains typically dragging-down in type. Chronic constipation with canine hunger is common and they are always better for quick, brisk movements as dancing or walking and worse for thunderstorms.

Sexual Problems

Difficulties are psychological in origin with few exceptions due to hormonal inbalance or as a complication of certain synthetic drug treatments — particularly the contraceptive 'pill' can frequently dampen libido. Often there is an underlying problem of immature distortion or ambivalence to the opposite sex, sometimes dating from earliest years. This needs to be discussed together with the whole area of sexual fantasy. Whenever possible, limit childish magical thinking and omnipotence by frank open discussion. There should be no 'secrets' about sex as these cluster together and only feed the problem areas. On the whole the response to homoeopathy in both sexes is very encouraging.

REMEDIES

For premature ejeculation *Nux Vomica, Lycopodium, Medorrhinum.*

For impotency, *Silicea, Selenium, Caladium, Arg, Nit.*
For frigidity, *Pulsatilla, Ignatia, Platina, Graphites, Onosmodium.*
For painful intercourse, *Causticum.*
For 'honeymoon' cystitis — *Staphisagria.*

Shingles (Herpes Zoster)

Infiltration of a spinal nerve root by the chicken pox virus in any part of the body and most common in elderly adults. There is pain, irritation, discomfort from the characteristic rash with vesticles and burning pain along the nerve-root distribution of the skin — usually on one side of the body. There may be prolonged severe neuralgic pain after the acute attack due to scarring of the vesticles on healing.

REMEDIES

Rhus Tox, Ranunculus Bulb, Sulphur, Arsenicum, Lachesis, Mezereum.

Silicea (Silica)

Trituration of the element. A deep acting polycrest remedy for chronic disease. The patient is typically thin and chilly, sweating profusely and offensively, especially about the feet which feel as if in a 'wet sock' most of the day. There is great exhaustion with nervousness and timidity — lacking totally in 'grit', confidence, the ability to see a problem through, or staying power and determination. There are many chronic problems of inflammation with pus formation. *Silicea* is often called the 'mother of pus', because every lesion seems to suppurate and discharge pus. Occipital headaches, radiating forward over the vertex to the forehead or over one eye. The skin is typically cracked and infected, the fingers dead white. Every symptom is aggravated by chill and the least cold draught of air. Enuresis.

Simillimum

The homoeopathic remedy that has the power in its original unpotentised toxic state to produce similar symptoms to those of the patient and thereby to relieve them by its action on the vital energy in this same area. According to Hahnemann the simillimum has a natural tendency to form similar symptoms as in its undiluted state and it is this tendency which allows the patient's symptoms to be unlocked and available to the normal process of resistance and cure which is intrinsic to everyone.

I personally feel that vital energy is bound by suppressed illness creating — suppressed energy and that the potencies are able to release this trapped, bound-up self or vital energy so that it can find a new and healthy level of expression and functioning again.

Simpson, Sir James Young (1811-1870)

The eminent Edinburgh professor of midwifery who first used — both in surgery and labour, chloroform as an anaesthetic. He was teacher and friend of Skinner and Drysdale. Although not a homoeopath, he nevertheless was in advance of his time in many major area. Particularly he advocated single-remedy prescribing rather than the poly-pharmacy of his time. He had a great influence over Skinner and paved the way for many of his later contributions. In homoeopathy single remedy prescribing is one of the major therapeutic principles.

Sinusitis

Inflammation of the mucous membrane of the sinuses, leading to catarrh, discharge and headache — often over one eye with local tenderness over the blocked sinus due to the inflammation.

REMEDIES
Pulsatilla, Hepar Sulph, Kali Bic, Sulphur.

Skinner, Thomas M.D. (1825-1906)

The distinguished Edinburgh homoeopath who until the age of fifty was antagonistic to the method — as indeed was at first Hering, and many other eminent early workers. He later practised in Liverpool and London, working closely with Clarke and Burnett.

His major work is *Homoeopathy and Gynæcology (1878).*

Sleep Problems

The common problem which often requires careful exploration and prescribing. The cause may vary from pain of arthritis, rheumatism, organic disease, nutritional abuse or an overactive mind due to temperament. Anxiety generally is a common cause.

Lycopodium 6— For an over-active mind, unable to rest or relax.
Aconitum — From fear and anxiety.
Coffea 6 — Due to abuse of tea or coffee.
Nux Vox 5 — From dietary indiscretions.
Arsenicum — Waking with fear and anxiety after midnight to 1.00 am.
Kali Carb.— Waking with anxiety in the early morning hours — 3-5.00 am.
Pulsatilla — Insomnia due to the heat of the bed.
Lachesis — From drenching night-sweats.

Sleep Walking (Somnambulism)

There is usually a deep underlying psychological problem that needs exploring when it is persistent.
REMEDIES
Kali Brom, Stramonium, Lycopodium.

Snoring

The common problem. The underlying causes need exploring including polyps, adenoids, chronic throat infections, catarrh.
REMEDIES
Opium 6, Kali Bic. 6.

Sol

Potentisation of lactose powders exposed to sunlight. Useful for problems aggravated by heat or the sun's rays with intolerence to sunlight of any kind as can occur in certain sensitive skin conditions or photophobia. Also indicated for sunstroke and allergies worse for heat and sun.

Solidago Virgo Aurea (Golden Rod)

A remedy for chronic conditions of the renal organs, particularly with low renal output and renal colic. Dysuria. Urinary retention, (compare *Natrum Mur* and *Causticum.*)

Spasm

Spasm can occur in any part of the body wherever there is smooth muscle. Symptoms are pain, interference with normal physiological functining and often anxiety. The cause may be fear, apprehension or in some cases irritation from physical factors — a calculus, dietary irritation or allergy.

REMEDIES

Aconitum, when due to fear. Spasm of the throat and glottis.

Drosera, Ignatia, Cicuta. Spasm of the larynx.

Causticum. Of the bronchial tubes.

Phosphorus, of the stomach.

Nux Vom. Of the calf muscles.

Cuprum Met.

Spigelia (Pinkroot)

Tincture of the whole plant. Mainly a left-side remedy. There is severe neuralgia of the face, neck and shoulders, aggravated by cold air, touch, or movement. (compare *Kalmia, Colchicum, Belladonna, Platina, Nux Vom.*) Also palpitations with Angina *(Cactus, Latrodectus).*

Spongia Tosta

An important cardiac remedy with anxiety, palpitations, fear of death, depression and cardiac pain. There may be valvular disease of the heart with shortness of breath, cardiac enlargement and weakness. Cardiac asthma. Laryngitis with hoarseness, dryness of the throat. All symptoms worse for sleep *(Lachesis)* and better for sitting up and warm drinks. The breathlessness is aggravated by lying flat.

Sprains

Traumatic injury to the tendons as a result of fall or strain. The tendons are stretched, bruised or torn in severe cases with characteristic pain, swelling, incapacity and stiffness. Swelling of the area may be marked due to haematoma.

REMEDIES

Arnica, Bellis, Perrenis, Calc. Carb, Kali Carb, Sulphur.

Stammering

The common stutter. A nervous problem of speech, mainly psychological in origin. It is always aggravated by any new situation or pressure of any kind.

REMEDIES

Belladonna, Mercurius, Stramonium. These often need to be combined with regular speech-therapy sessions, especially in severe cases.

Stannum (Tin)

There is increasing weakness, weight-loss and exhaustion. In general the patient is withdrawn and has no interest due to a near-collapsed general state. Typically pale with severe neuralgia and laryngeal hoarseness — there is chronic catarrh with thick, yellowish mucous discharge. Leucorrhoea, the discharge thick creamy-yellow.

Stapf, Ernest, M.D. (1788-1860)

The German homoeopath, born in Nurenburg who was the earliest of Hahnemann's pupils and disciple thoughout his life. He was also a close friend of Quin. He studied and worked in homoeopathy as early as 1811, assisting Hahnemann with the *Materia Medica Pura* and working with the limited repertory of the early days. Like Hahnemann, he was both ridiculed and often persecuted by his colleagues for his viewpoint — although later considered to be a most respected and serious physician. He was one of the earliest provers of Hahnemann's original group and worked with him in proving some 32 remedies. He became founder and first editor of the very first homoeopathic journal in the world — Archiv. fur die Homopathirsche Heilkunst — 1822-39. A staunch believer in the harmful effects to the patient of coffee, wine, and tobacco, he may have been the first appointed royal homoeopathic physician. In 1835 he became visiting physician to the royal household, having previously carried out homoeopathic treatments by letter.

His major works include:

Additions to the Materia Medica Pura (1846).

Staphysagria (Stavesacre)

One of the our most valuable remedies wherever there is anger or irritability with indignation and buried resentments. Pain is present — severe, tearing and stitch-like. Cystitis from trauma or injury with bruising, prostrate problems. Impotence. Especially useful after surgery for pain around the incision. Unconscious resentment and anger afterwards is always characteristic.

Sterility

This is a major and often complex problem which needs careful and thorough medical investigation to ascertain the causes. They may lie with either partner and it is important to know the roots of the problem and whether there is scarring of the tubes from earlier infection or if the sperm count is low — as may follow adult mumps.

REMEDIES

For chronic scarring and blockage of the fallopian tubes following infection or operation include *Silica, Graphites, Thiosinaminum.* For diminished sperm count consider *Sepia, Silicea, Lycopodium.* It is important that the homoeopath works closely with a gynaecologist colleague in most cases.

Sticta (Lungwort)

Tincture of the fresh plant. It acts primarily upon mucous membrane of the respiratory tract with bronchial catarrh. The nasal secretions are dry and typically difficult to expel with little secretion. There are recurrent colds and chronic rheumatic problems. All symptoms are worse for lying down and often aggravated during the night.

Stonham, Thomas M.D. (1858-1903)

The homoeopathic physician and co-author of *Manual of Homoeo-therapeutics.*

Storage of homoeopathic remedies

Homoeopathic remedies keep indefinitely without losing strength or efficacy provided that they are always stored in a dry, cool, air-tight glass container. This is infinitely preferable to plastic storage bottles, because of chemical impurities present in such containers. The glass bottles should always be thoroughly clean and not have been used to store either homoeopathic or conventional remedies in the past. They should be stored away from any substance which could neutralise them, in particular camphor, menthol or strong perfume.

Stramonium (Thorn Apple)

Recommended for states of acute mental excitement, confusion, delirium with loss of control or voilent tendencies. There is manic excitement with a tendency to destructive impulses. Delusional beliefs with hallucinations. Convulsions — epileptic or hysterical. Puerperal psychosis with violence and acute mania. Suicidal impulses. Stroke, loss of consciousness. Meningitis with excitement or restlessness are the other characteristics.

Stroke

The acute cerebral catastrophe — usually due to either cerebral haemorrhage, cerebral spasm or thrombosis. There is frequently loss of consciousness with a fixed dilated pupil, heavy, snoring, breathing and weakness of one limb. Often there is a history of raised blood pressure. Medical care is essential, sometimes hospitalisation.
REMEDIES
Arnica, Rescue Remedy, *Opium, Strmonium, Aconitum.*

Strophanthus Hispidus (Kombe Seed)

The remedy indicated for mainly cardiac irregularity with a variable pulse, palpitations and shortness of breath on effort. Especially of value where there is a history of chronic smoking or alcoholism (*Nux Vom*).

Styes

The common localised infection of the eyelids — either acute and clearing completely, or recurrent. In some cases it is a chronic condition the stye remaining for many months and never really better. Irritation is its main feature.
REMEDIES
Pulsatilla, Staphisagria, Hepar Sulph, Calc. Carb, Baryta Carb, Silicea.

233

Suicidal Impulses

Suicidal thoughts of a passing nature are very common and usually no more than a temporary idea and dramatic fantasy which is never acted upon or seriously considered. Suicide is always an act ·of aggression and in some cultures the most aggressive act conceivable is to commit suicide on an enemy's doorstep. It is not unfortunately rare in our culture and the thought may become a threat and a reality when part of a depressive illness. In severe depression, such fantasies become realities and threats must always be taken seriously and preferably under the care or wing of a physician having a good rapport and understanding with the patient and a natural sympathy for the problem. If anyone reading this book at this moment is desperate and isolated they can obtain help by contacting by phone the nearest branch of The Samaritans — at any time — day or night. Their address is in the telephone book or the operator will give it to you.

REMEDIES
Aurum Met, Arg Nit, Alumina, Capsicum, Naja, Natrum Mur, Natrum Sulph, Nux. Vom.

Sulphur (Flowers of Sulphur)

The most important of Hahnemann's anti-psora remedies for chronic disease. Body-shape is varied, but frequently thin, bent-over, red-faced, untidy and unhealthy-looking. They take little exercise being chronically tired and exhausted. Always intolerant of heat they are warm-blooded and need few clothes or covering on the coldest day. The skin is typically unhealthy and infected with a variety of discharging sores and rashes often of a thick, offensive nature. Morning diarrhoea typically drives them out of bed and is also offensive. They crave fats, but water or bathing aggravates. There are flashes of heat with hot-flushes, drenching sweats and weariness. The mind is full of plans and projects, but always unrealisable or unrealistic and rarely carried through to a conclusion. It is a remedy for chronic problems where there is little or no response to well-indicated homoeopathic prescribing.

Sulphuric Acid

A remedy for depression combined with exhaustion and near-collapse. The patient is restless and in a hurry (*Medorrhinum*). Tremor is part of the weakness, and chronic skin problems occur because of reduced vitality. Boils, bed-sores, ulceration, chronic indigestion. A sore cracked mouth is characteristic, ulcerated and infected at the corners with bleeding (cp. *Silicea, Nitric Ac.*). Pyorrhoea, the gums unhealthy, often infected contibutes to depression and lowering of resistance. Mainly a right-sided remedy.

Sunstroke

This can be a very dangerous or fatal condition when exposure has been severe or prolonged in a sensitive person. The exposure may have been to the sun's rays or to heat generally — both of which can be perilous if excessive. Symptoms are throbbing, headache, weakness, collapse, vomiting, redness and loss of consciousness with fits or paralysis. Hospitalisation is essential in severe cases.

REMEDIES

Glonoin, Aconitum, Belladonna, Pulsatilla, Bryonia. Repeat the remedy every few minutes until there is a vital response.

Suppression

In any form — suppression of person, opinion or symptoms is against basic homoeopathic principle and practise. The only exception is that of an overwhelming infection, after an operation — when pain is severe and unbearable or in terminal illness, and even in the latter — only pain and not awareness should be blocked. Homoeopathy anticipated psychoanalytic insight by nearly a century when it warned against the dangers of suppression. It can never lead to cure and at best only relieves for temporary periods. Suppression of symptoms, means suppression of vital response, of energy and ultimately the person. Many of our major modern conventional synthetic drugs act totally by this means — suppressing reactions, natural response and resistance, particularly the steriod group, the tranquillisers, anti-depressants and antibiotics. The worst offender is the steroid, now frequently prescribed for the most benign, superficial eczema from the first weeks of life and continued intermittently — sometimes for years as the original condition becomes chronic and never fully cured. Suppression of symptoms never gets to the roots of a condition or the cause of an illness — either physical or psychological. In general the problem is quite simply driven 'underground' where it festers, becomes chronic and is in danger of re-appearing in a new, more resistant form, sometimes in a deeper organ or quite new area of the body and this time much more difficult to treat. Homoeopathy aims at stimulating the vital reation of the individual and the organism overall to the full, seeing this as the only true and curative pathway for treatment and cure. Suppression over the years is one of the major causes of chronic disease in our society and is a recipe for disaster.

Swann, Dr. (–   )

The American homoeopath and innovator who first prepared the nosode *Lyssin* from the saliva of a rabid dog as a prophylactic treatment for rabies. He worked with Fincke, Grimmer, Bach and Wheeler on the nosodes and is generally known for his work on the high potencies. He described a first proving of *Lueticum* in 1880. He also developed the nosode *Anthracium* from anthrax and a *Tuberculinum* nosode from tuberculosis sputum.

Sycosis (Fig-Wart disease)

One of the three major miasms of chronic disease postulated by Hahnemann. It is thought to be due to previously suppressed gonorrhoeal illness acting as an inherited sub-clinical parasite to the body, undermining health, resistance and energy. The major clinical symptoms are in the skin and take the form of multiple cauliflower-like warts, having a stalk or a root, and particularly common in the anal-gential area. Chill on the warmest day is characteristic. *Thuja* is the major sycotic remedy for this miasm, with *Nitric Acid* next in importance.

Sycotic Co. (Paterson)

The bowel nosode. This is a catarrhal remedy acting on mucous membrane throughout the body. Irritability is the key-note mentally, also of the mucous and synovial membranes. Pale, puffy under the eyes and anaemic looking, nervous tension is characteristic together with a variety of catarrhal symptoms anywhere in the body. There are digestive difficulties, diarrhoea, conjunctivitis, nasal catarrh, deafness, tonsillitis or sore throat. Asthma or cystitis with painful spasms, or other renal irritations as nephritis or pyelitis. The angles of the mouth, nose and anal area are often cracked, sore and ulcerated. The tongue is fissured. Leucorrhoea. Aversion to eggs.

Symphocarpus Racemosa (Snowberry)

Tincture of the fresh berries. A remedy for severe retching and nausea — as vomiting of pregnancy, sometimes constant throught the day and night. There is complete lack of interest in food.

Symphytum (Comfrey)

The ancient remedy for deep-seated pains of bones from whatever cause and of assistance whenever there is delay in healing and uniting of fractures.

Symptoms

That which is experienced by the patient personally as the expression of his malaise. All symptoms are seen by the homoeopath as ultimately a healthy vital reaction and struggle towards balance and the individual response to underlying inbalance and dis-ease. Symptoms are not however the cause of the illness, but only the visible external manifestation of internal malaise, dating back over several weeks or months. Absence or weakness of symptom-response is of more concern to the homoeopath than its presence, reflecting severely limited resistance and vitality. Symptoms are the body's attempts to regain homoeostasis and cure and this quite vital reaction-of-cure needs conserving. It is the underlying meaning of the symptoms that needs treatment rather than the symptoms themselves and simple eradication is undesirable and not in the patient's best long-term interests. Homoeopathy takes an overall viewpoint and totality of symptoms into account when prescribing.

Symptomatic Treatment

The treatment and relief of symptoms only by conventional allopathic means is short-term thinking and only rarely justifiable. The short-term gain does nothing to understand or treat underlying causes and is a major factor in recurrent disease and the need for constant re-prescribing. Stronger remedies have the dual danger of side-effects and suppression-of-symptoms at the expense of cure.

Syncope (fainting)

The common problem of loss of consciousness for a brief time — often from emotional causes and sometimes recurrent.

REMEDIES

Pulsatilla — for recurrent fainting at the least emotional situation or from heat.

Aconitum — when the attack is provoked by fear.

Ignatia — when due to emotion and especially from grief and loss or fear of it.

China — For fainting at the sight of blood.

Veratrum Alb — from pain or emotion — the patient deathly pale in a cold sweat and seemingly about to succumb.

Give the remedy in the 6th potency every few minutes until recovery occurs. A few drops of the potency in water on the tongue is the most convenient form of application for syncope.

Syphilinum

The syphilis nosode prepared by lysis of infected serous exudate of the primal chancre and made into potency by serial dilutions. First suggested by Lux in 1830. Swann carried out the initial provings and published the results fifty years later in 1880. The main indications are chronic conditions, sometimes with a history of miscarriage. Failure to thrive, and chronic varicose ulcers. Mental symptoms are marked with devious avoidance-behaviour towards others which may take a phobic form with fear of contact, infection and germs. They are noisy, difficult, stubborn at times, tearful, opposing, varying in mood but especially prone to obsessional hand-washing, mannerisms, tics and movements.

Insomnia is characteristic, with all symptoms worse at night or for sea air (*Nat. Mur*). There is typical pain in the tibia or long bones, often in the night with a thin, prematurely aged look. The teeth are poor, deformed, notched and cracked or 'Peg' type. Arteriosclerosis, urinary weakness, impotency, genital itching. Problems of pruritis, leucorrhoea — greenish and offensive. Chronic exhaustion with depression.

Tabacum (Tobacco)

Tincture of the fresh plant. A remedy for nausea with pallor, cold sweats and prostration. Travel sickness, pregnancy sickness, convulsions, oedema of the soft palate. Vertigo. All symptoms worse for heat (*Pulsatilla*) and better for lying down, darkness and sleep.

Tachycardia

Increase in heart rate. The normal pulse rate is 72 beats per minute. In tachycardia the rate is increased to 150 or 200 beats per minute. Causes include emotion, infection with fever, toxic or poisonous causes, excesses of tea or coffee, other stimulant drugs, allergy, side-effects of drugs, degeneration.
REMEDIES
Lycopus Virg., Spigelia, Crataegus, Tarantula Hisp.

Taking the remedies

The homoepathic medicine is mainly on the surface of the tablet or pill. It is important that whenever possible they should not be handled except to a minimum in order to avoid neutralising them by any perfume or foodstuff on the hands, or by handling generally. Similarly homoeopathic remedies should be taken away from food, either before or after unless there are specific instructions to this effect from the physician. Strong food or drink including coffee, tea, mint, alcohol, should not be taken within half an hour of the remedy.

Tamus Communis (Black Bryony)

One of the most powerful remedies for chillblains with painful itching and redness. It is often used in low potency or as mother tincture.

Tapeworm

The solitary parastic worm intestinal condition, now relatively rare due to improved hygiene and preventative practise. Its origin is from infected uncooked beef or pork. Symptoms are abdominal pain, weight-loss and segments of the worm in the stool. Isolated causes can still occur and careful diagnosis is essential.

REMEDIES
Calc. Carb, Spigelia, Sulphur, Sabadilla, Sepia, Silicea.

Tarantula Cubensis (Cuben Tarantula)

Severe burning pains with abscess formation and collapse. Anthrax infection. The face is violet or there is pallor, cold sweating, a sinking sensation with emaciation, shortness of breath and air hunger. Both legs and ankles are swollen. Shock — a remedy for the most desperate conditions with lack of response or vitality of reaction. (*Carbo Veg, Veratrum Alb.*)

Tarantula Hisp (Spanish Tarantula)

A remedy for states of severe violent restlessness and destructive behaviour — impulsive and anxious in the extreme. There are burning pains of the limbs with weakness. Also similar symptoms in the rectum and anus. Over-sensitive to the least stimulus, all symptoms are aggravated by cold and damp. Indicated in severe mental conditions of hysteria, pyschosis, manic excitment. Bright colours and music often aggravate symptoms. Destructiveness and tearing of clothes is frequent, jerking movements of the head, agitiation, chronic indigestion, flatulence. Shooting pains of the uterus and vagina. Diarrhoea with blood, spasms of the bladder, prostatis, pruritis, palpitations. The pulse is rapid and irregular.

The key-note is irritation, congestion, burning pains of any part of the body with severe uncontrollable impulses to violence.

Taraxacum Officinalis (Dandelion, 'Pee-in-the-bed')

Its main indications are hepititis — the liver enlarged and tender, deficient in functioning. They are intolerant of any form of touch. Enuresis.

Taste — loss of

May frequently accompany a severe cold or 'flu, with associated nasal catarrh and throat congestion affecting the mucosa and inhibiting the taste sensitivity of the tongue's surface. In some cases the condition may become chronic.

REMEDIES

Natrum Mur — following cold or flu,

Merc Sol — the tongue dirty and offensive with thick yellow coating,

Pulsatilla — when due to general congestion — everything has an earthy-like taste to it,

Nux Vom, — with a generalised sour acid taste whatever is taken, worse in the morning, the tongue has a thick white coating, aggravated by alochol or smoking,

Calcarea — for chronic problems everything tastes generally sour and unpalatable,

Sulphur another chronic remedy for loss of taste the food tastes either vinegary or of blood.

Teeth

Thorough regular cleaning and flossing are essential for healthy teeth together with dental hygiene and regular prophylactic check-ups to ensure that problems are detected early or avoided. The diet and quality of nuitrition is often the key to healthy dental development and sweet, sugary and refined foods should be avoided whenever possible and shown to be undesirable rather than given as rewards to the young. Decayed or badly-placed teeth blocking the emergence of new ones must be removed. Root abscess must be drained whenever present because of the narrowness of the dental canal and dangers of abscess formation and spread of infection. It should not be just sealed-off under a dressing and local antibiotic before the pus has fully drained from the area.

REMEDIES
For caries and unhealthy dental development include *Silicea, Calc. Carb., Phosphorus, Calc. Phos, Kreosotum.* Often the constitutional prescription is required to stimulate healthier growth and vitality.

Teething Problems of the infant

The commonest symptoms are irritability, gum soreness, the child wanting something in the mouth all the time to bite upon. Problems are most acute from the age of a year when the 4 bicuspids emerge after the incisors.

REMEDIES
Chamomilla 30, — the child irritable and dislikes being put down,
Aconitum where there is fear and restless agitation,
Belladonna with red face, temperature and crying when examined or touched,
Cina is useful where an irritating cough is associated,
Drosera when the cough is dry and goes on to vomiting,
Merc Sol. should be considered for a child covered in sweat and with profuse, offensive salivation.
Calc Carb. When teething is retarded, along with all the milestones especially for a flabby child with forehead sweating.

Tellurium

Introduced by Hering in 1850. A remedy to consider for chronic skin problems especially ringworm of the face and body. Chronic infection is everywhere with pusy discharge (*Sulphur*). Middle ear infection with a thick offensive purulent discharge. Sweating is offensive (*Silicea*). There is intolerence of the least touch or pressure.

Tendonitis

The inflammatory condition of painful tendons after strain or excessive unaccustomed usage. Swelling, pain, spasm, aching with a bruised sensation is common. Rest, firm strapping or support, avoidance of fatigue in the area affected together with the appropriate remedy usually clears the condition in a few days. Local heat is often beneficial.

REMEDIES

Rhus Tox 6, Arnica.

Tension States

The common psychological state of anxiety, restlessness, muscular tension, aching, pains, spasm of stomach or back, palpitations. Panic, exaggeration and distortion of any reality problems is also present. Discussion and the free-expression of a particular area of anxiety is essential although often there is nothing specific to resolve and the tension is a re-emergence of long-standing problems. In all cases physical symptoms of diarrhoea or indigestion need careful attention to exclude an organic problem and must always form part of the totality when selecting the remedy. A psychological state should never be prescribed for on the mentals alone without considering the physical state.

REMEDIES

Natrum Mur, Arsenicum, Lycopodium, Gelsemium, Ignatia, Pulsatilla, Sepia.

Terebinth (Oil of Turpentine)

Tincture of the rectified oil. Predominately a kidney remedy, there are severe unbearable burning pains with irritation, haematuria (blood in the urine), dragging, weight-like pains in the kidney area as from nephritis. Cystitis with strangury (pain and spasm at the end of the urinary flow). Little urine is passed. There is generalised congestion of mucous membrane throughout the body with irritation in the areas affected. The remedy is closely related to *Thuja, Cantharis, Berberis, Cannabis Sat.,* and careful comparison is essential.

Terrain of the Patient

The 'soil' or terrain of the patient refers to the concept fundamental to homoeopathy — that all illness is a combination of diseased physiology with increased susceptibility and diminished resistance and vital energy. The usual 'cause' of disease is a miasm in chronic disease, or from such internal irritants as toxins, parasites or anything that undermines healthy functioning of the part affected. Bacteria, mites, tics and viral agents are seen as the natural symbiotic inhabitants of our overall environment which only when the terrain is weakened and made more susceptible, no longer live in symbiosis with us. Under such conditions they may then actively invade and undermine tissue-functioning leading to infection, inflammation, tumor or abscess formation, but only after the physiological terrain has been previously undermined and un-balanced. One of the major undermining factors is undoubtedly that of psychological stress or shock with dietary neglect or abuse, coming a close second. Stress can lower the healthy sperm count of the most virile donor within hours — such is its depth of action on vitality generally.

Terminal Conditions

The homoeopathic remedy often has an important role to play in terminal conditions and can relieve or lessen symptoms and their effects upon the patient's peace of mind. It can 'smooth the way', and allow a patient to die with dignity, yet retain awareness and peace of mind. The homoeopathic remedy is not curative here and because of lack of vital energy there is usually a poor response to the 'local' 6c or 3x potencies. It is the higher potencies which are most valuable, especially the 30 and 200. These can often make the patient wonderfully calm, serene and relaxed so that they need far less pain-killers and opiates. Tension, anticipation and worry is also relieved.

In some cases the higher potencies have given a marked, albeit temporary relief from all symptoms for a period of several weeks or months. Naturally this cannot occur in every case or even often and each case must be seen according to its unique picture, the extent and length of time of the illness — in short, every case be treated homoeopathically.

Teste, Alphonse, M.D. (1814-1988)

The French homoeopath who published in 1844 *A Practical Manual of Animal Magnetism,* containing an exposition of the methods employed in the producing magnetic phenomena and its application to the treatment and cure of disease. Translated by Dr. Spillan. In 1854 he wrote *The Homoeopathic Materia Medica,*

Arranged by Systems, (Tr. Hempe). Also *A Homoepathic Treatise of Diseases of Children.*

Testicular Problems

These should always be treated by the physician to ensure careful diagnosis and treatment. The common problem of undescended testicle must be corrected either homoeopathically or surgically if the potencies fail to elicit a positive response.

REMEDIES

Pulsatilla, Aurum Met.

Hydrocoele or fluid around the testicular sac, is a less urgent problem and seen quite commonly. The origin is sometimes associated with an earlier history of tuberculosis.

REMEDIES

Pulsatilla, Tub. Bov.

Orchitis or inflammation of the testicle may be a complication of mumps — one of the commoner causes.

REMEDIES

The mumps nosode *Parotidinum, Merc. Sol, Spongia Tost, Pulsatilla, Thuja.*

Tetanus

Severe infection leading to septicaemia, which may follow tetanus contamination of a dirty wound or fracture. The wound must be carefully cleaned with *Calendula* and any foreign material removed. When in doubt, or the wound heavily contaminated with soil or dirty foreign matter give the specific anti-tetanus vaccine.

REMEDIES

Ledum, Hypericum, Arnica, Merc. Sol, Cicuta Virosa.

Teucrium (Timothy Grass)

For hay fever where there is sensitivity to grass pollens. Indicated as prophylactic in early cases.

Theridion (The orange spider of Curacao)

Oversensitivity and excitement to any stimulus with hysterical behaviour or depression. All symptoms are aggravated by noise including the chronic nausea and severe pains. Emanciation with loss of weight. Fainting, chill and headache from the forehead backwards towards the base of the skull. Worse for the least noise. Turberculosis, chronic catarrh, morning sickness from gastric catarrah. Nausea of pregnacy and emotional origin. Seasickness, weakness, impotence are other major indicators.

Threadworms

Common in children, infection with the minute threadworm can spread throughout the family and frequently involve the parents who also present with the typical symptoms of anal irritation, worse at night. Often the fine white, cotton-wool threadworms can be seen on the stools to confirm the diagnosis and the condition has been recently presently treated in one of the children. Another common symptom is itching of the nose. In the child there is also irritation, insomnia, crying during sleep, gritting the teeth, weight-loss, appetite-loss, vomiting with thirst. There is nearly always increased general nervousness. In all cases the nails should be carefull cut back short and kept scrupously clean. Personal hygiene must be at a high level to avoid constant re-infection.

REMEDIES

Cina 30 for nasal and anal irritation,
Aconitum for the very earliest cases,
Merc. Sol for long-standing problems, resistant to cure,
Nux Vom is indicated for teeth-grinding at night.
Belladonna is helpful to the night-terrors or nightmares.

Thlaspi Pursa Pastoris (Pasteur's Purse)

An unusual remedy, indicated for disordered menstrual conditions where there is intermittent flow — the periods occuring on alternative months.

Throat Sore

The condition may be involve the soft tissues at the back of the throat causing pharyngitis or be more forward with inflammation of the vocal chords so that there is Laryngitis with hoarseness. See specific headings.

The condition may be less localised and non-specific due to cold or flu, sometimes over-use of the throat and voice.

REMEDIES

Aconitum for acute cases, with restless fever, anxiety and a burning sensation in the throat,

Belladonna is for similar conditions, the throat bright-red, the patient motionless and worse for swallowing.

Merc. Sol for severe infections with pus formation and profuse sweating,

Phytolacca has a sore purple throat unable to swallow,

Lachesis is similar but often left-sided.

Consider also *Bryonia, Pulsatilla, Natrum Mur, Arnica* — the latter for strain from over-use.

Thrush

Infection with the herpes virus and increasingly a cause of chronic problems involving mucous membrane of the eyes, throat and genital regions in particular. It can also invade surrounding skin areas with outcrops of herpes vesticles in the active phase. It is highly infectious, affects both sexes and causes varied symptoms as sore throat, leucorrhoea, cystitis. The condition may be sexually transmitted but many cases are caused by the more ordinary contact. The disease is resistant to most conventional treatments and chronic cases are commonly seen by the homoeopath.

REMEDIES

Sulphur, Nitric Ac. A constitutional prescription is often required.

Thuja Occidentalis (Tree of Life)

Hahnemann's major remedy for sycotic miasm states of chronic disease. The typical make-up is usually thin and unhealthy-looking, wasted with profuse offensive sweating over the whole body. Fig-warts and excrescences of hands, feet and especially anal-gential region are characteristic, with a tendency to itch, split or bleed in the area affected. There may be flatter, multiple brownish warts or markings. Shingles with vesicle formation and post-shingles neuralgic pains. For illness that has commenced after vaccination. Bladder problems and cystitis, urethritis, ovarian pain on ovulation. The mental state is one of irritability. Delusional bizarre ideas, jealousy (*Lachesis*). Odd convictions that the body is made of glass and will break. Of a live animal in the abdomen, or headaches — as if a nail has been driven through the skull because the pain is so localised.

Thyroidinum (Thyroid extract)

For slow retarded states with fluid retention and oedema. Exopthalmic goitre (protrusion of the eyeballs). Chronic constipation, heart disability especially angina, tachycardia. The skin is dry and cool. Psoriasis. Alopoecia. Nocturnal enuresis. Fibroid tumours of the breast or uterus. Heavy periods.

Tics

The common psychological nervous problem with involuntary movements of any part of the body, aggravated by an unfamiliar situation or increase of psychological pressure. 'Live flesh' or tics around the lower eyelid are common to most people at some time where there has been a build-up of tension or fatigue — the body unable to 'let go' or relax adequately. Patient discussion, reassurance and sometimes specialised help to understand the mechanism and gains or function of the symptom may be necessary when severe or shronic.
REMEDIES
Natrum Mur., Nux Vom., Agaricus, Arsenicum.

Time Modalities

Certain remedies, especially the broader and deeper-acting polycrests have a time of day or night when they are most active with typical aggravation of symtoms. Knowledge of such modalities, linked to the physiological clock, have a value in prescribing and give a check on accuracy. Examples are — *Arsenicum* — midnight to 1.00 am., *Kali Carb.* 3.00-5.00 am., *Lycopodium* 4.00-8.00 am. *Nat. Mur* 9.00-11.00 am.

Tongue — problems of

The condition of the tongue, its general appearance and health have always given an important clue to the overall state of individual health. A thick-coated tongue may indicate chronic

252

digestive problems and a remedy as *Nux Vom*. A thick but more white coating indicates *Bryonia*. Where the coating is yellow and offensive, consider *Mercurius*. Inflammation and ulceration may come from traumatic causes — the tongue bitten in an accident or a convulsion. Give *Arnica*. Where the sides of the tongue are painful and swollen as after an insect bite, use *Apis*. An acute infection or glossitis may require *Belladonna* if the tongue is bright red and burning with pain and discomfort. Where the redness and burning is at the tip, use *Rhus Tox*.

Tonsillitis

Inflammation of the tonsil with pain, raised temperature, swelling tender local lymph glands of the neck region. Exhaustion, vomiting and severe discomfort is common and swallowing is usually painful. For abscess in this area see section Quinsy.

REMEDIES
Aconitum, Baryta Carb, Belladonna, Phytolacca, Sulphur, Hepar Sulph, Silicea, Merc. Sol.

Toothache

Pain from dental caries, sometimes due to root abscess with cheek tenderness. Dental examination and treatment is needed in all cases. See other heading — Teeth problems.

REMEDIES
For acute toothache *Aconitum, Coffea, Chamomilla, Nux Vom, Belladonna, China, Staphisagria, Plantago, Spigelia, Mag. Carb, Selenium.*

Torticollis (Wry neck)

The common condition of stiff neck, usually rheumatic in origin from exposure to chill, cold air or draught, provoking spasm of local muscles. It is nearly always short-lasting and usually clears up spontaneously in a few days with warmth, protection and the appropriate remedy. If it fails to resolve quickly, it may by psychological in origin or from a different deeper cause which needs proper investigating.

REMEDIES
Natrum Mur, Nux Vom, Arg. Nit, Causticum, Dulcamara, Merc. Sol.

Totality of the approach

The basis of all homoeopathy. In the Organon (para. 7), Hahnemann describes the totality of symptoms as the outer image of the individual only, reflecting the inner essence of the disease and disturbed the vital (life) force. Totality of approach takes into account both of these — the symptoms and the inner depths and considerations and detailed appraisal of all the symptoms but includes the causative factors, the patient's aura or relationship with the doctor and rapport established. It should take into account the spoken as well as the unspoken communications, the subjective as well as the objective impressions, presentation, appearance, expressions and associations. Especially the mind with all the feelings, motivations, pains and attitudes are vital and relevent. Also the type of work, clothes, the gait, body-odour, mannerisms each and every aspect — both physical and mental contributes to an overall totality of impression and fact. The majority of the patient's symptoms must fit the remedy and odd isolated symptoms can be ignored once they have been carefully considered in the diagnostic process. The concept of totality expresses a whole — a hypothesis, including the symptoms, the simillimum, the cause which may be grief, stress, shock, trauma, loss, suppression, miasm, so that eventually the totality comes to express far more than its component parts taken in isolation.

Tracheitis

Inflammation of the trachea. The common upper respiratory tract infection with soreness and pain. Often raw in type with cough, raised temperature, hoarseness and laryngitis also present, It is a frequent complication of the common cold and needs careful treatment to avoid pulmonary involvement as bronchitis.
REMEDIES
Aconitum, Bryonia, Belladonna, Sulphur, Mercurius, Hepar Sulph.

Travel Sickness

The problem of motion sickness. Especially a difficulty of the young, it can occur at any age. See heading Sea-Sickness. It is common in the sensitive nervous child in a car or bus and always aggravated by reading. Nausea, sweating, salivation, vomiting are common with a general sense of malaise.

REMEDIES

Cocculus, Pulsatilla, Natrum Mur, Nux Vom.

Treatment — aims of homoeopathic

In all cases, the aim is simply and solely to restore the person to full normal balance and health. The symptoms or dis-ease manifestations are not the prime concern of the homoeopath, nor should they be for the patient. Symptoms are indications and guide-lines — pointers to prescribe only and should not distract the homoeopath away from restoring vital energy and well-being, at deepest levels to the patient. Once this deep level is restored and corrected, then the external manifestations fall into place and perspective as vital energy flows and functions again.

Trillium Pendulum (White Beth-Root)

Primarily a gynaecolgical remedy, especially indicated for uterine haemorrhage and recurrent miscarriage of the third month. It has also a valuable role in menopausal flooding and fibroids.

Trituration

The unique process discovered by Hahnemann of making soluable for dilution and potency homoeopathic substances normally considered insoluble. Examples are *Silicea, Aurum Met*, or any of the other metals or minerals. During the initial titration the substance is mixed and ground up with lactose powder. This process is repeated — mixing and grinding until the substance becomes soluble — usually at the third trituration. Each tritutation is considered a centisimal-equivalent and the next dilution and succession in liquid forms as the 4th. centisimal potency.

Tuberculinum (Tub Bov.)

The subject of a detailed monogram and research by Compton-Burnett and one of his most important contributions. The nosode is prepared from tuberculous glandular material of infected cattle. It is a most important remedy acting deeply on problems of chronic disease which no other remedy can fully reach. There is a typical dry, hard, irritating, recurrent cough, intermittent fever with pallor, weight-loss and fainting. Often a history of T.B. infection either earlier or in a blood-relative. They are restless, love to travel and movement. The eye white or sclera often has a bluish tinge and period problems are frequent with nausea, migraines, sweating and great desire for fresh open air (*Pulsatilla*).

Tyler, Sir Henry James (1849-1910)

The eminent homoepath born Woodhull N.Y. Father of Dr. Margaret Tyler. He was benefactor to the London Homoeopathic Hospital in many generous ways creating the annual Tyler scholarship for studies to the U.S.A. Both Weir and Clarke were able to take advantage of such scholarships and studied with Hering and other contempories, widening their knowledge to the benefit of homoeopathy generally.

Tyler, Margaret, M.D. (1857-1943)

Daughter of Sir Henry Tyler, she worked tirelessly for the cause of homoeopathy for over 40 years at the London Homoeopathic Hospital. She was an inspired teacher and lecturer and by the Sir Henry Tyler scholarship — both she and her mother, were responsible for the transatlantic links and training of many of our earliest teachers with James Tyler Kent in Chicago. Despite opposition, she gave full support for high-potency prescribing and the single remedy. As a physician she was totally dedicated to her work, patients and students. Her major tour de force in writing was *Drug Pictures* (1942), which is still standard reading for present day students. She was editor of Homoeopathy from 1932-42. Author of an important paper on *Drosera,* she also wrote a correspondence course in homoeopathy for doctors unable to attend the lectures and formal courses at the hospital. She was particularly interested in the problem of the mentally handicapped subnormal child and held special clinics for these problems, working closely with the N.S.P.C.C.

Typhoid disease

Although in the past homoeopathy has played an important valuable role in the treatment of typhoid, I think that most colleagues would agree that the place of homoeopathy should be that of a secondary supportive treatment. It is far better to use modern antibiotics when available for the condition because of the often extreme virulence of the disease and dangers to the patient. The vital energy is often unable to rally when faced with such a severe attack and risks should never be taken for the sake of proving a principle. For the sake of completeness only , I am including some of the major remedies which can benefit the condition but in general Typhoid disease should be treated medically and in hospital.

REMEDIES

Remedies which have proved of value in the past are *Arsenicum, Baptisia, Bryonia, Carbo Veg, Ant. Crud, China, Croton Tig, Phosphoric Ac, Nux Vom.*

Typhus Fever

The highly infective .tic-born fever is also best dealt with by antibiotics — again because of its virulence and danger to the patient, particularly the young, with homoeopathy playing a supportive role in convalescant stages. Again for the sake of completeness only and where hospital or medical treatment is not immediately available. I am listing some of the principle remedies which may be indicated.

REMEDIES

Arsenicum, Carbo Veg, Agaricus, Sulphur.

Ulcer, Peptic

One of the commonest diseases of our time. As man increasingly lives in an environment where we have refined both ideals and food, cut off from root-origins and often family life, isolated from the meaning and end-result of work and insensitive to spiritual values, so he pays the penalty in terms of overall general health, especially of the stomach and digestive system. Having created a void for himself, man fills it with meaningless activities, often these take the form of tension and anxiety. Not only does nature abhor a vacuum, so too does the psyche and it rushes to fill it with fantasy, insecurity and often fear. All of this takes its toll in terms of peace of mind, essential for healthy digestion to occur. Acidity, flatulence, burning-pains, hot-air bubbles of wind, burping are all the expressions of inner stress and strain. Rushed instant meals are swallowed unchewed and washed down unsavoured. At other times, phases of over-eating and over-drinking starve the body of vitality in an attempt to survive the excesses. All of this combines to create an ulcer 'climate' with acidity or deep pain radiating to the shoulder blades, back or shoulder. The ulcer may cure spontaneously and completely without further symptoms or in others there is scar-tissue formed which creates further problems of narrowing, blockage and malfunctioning. In every case there is a risk of haemorrhage as an artery in the base of the ulcer becomes eroded. This may produce either the vomiting of fresh blood or its presence in the stools as undigested blood, the stool, black and tarry in appearance. Both are serious and may indicate the need

261

for surgery. A chronic ulcer which has been neglected for many years may become cancerous.

Whenever possible an ulcer should be prevented at an early stage by a reasoned, balanced, rhythmic life-style at all levels and an overall philosophy. When ulceration occurs, it should be treated as early as possible.

REMEDIES
Ornithogalum, Arg. Nit. (bleeding), *Nux Vom, Kali Carb, Arsenicum, Sulphur, Phosphorus* (bleeding).

Ulcer — varicose

The common complication of long-standing varicose veins, usually occuring at the ankle associated with obesity or chronic constipation. Ankle oedema and varicose eczema may be present and not infrequently there is a history of recurrent ulceration. An acute cause may be trauma of the ankle area of scratching from irritation. Treatment includes rest, elevation of the limb and leg exercises to stimulate the circulation. The ulcer should be cleaned with *Calendula* and kept covered with a dry sterile dressing. When infected and discharging pus, cover the ulcerated area with *Calendula* or honey and change the dressing after 3 days. Repeat the procedure until the pus has cleared.

REMEDIES
Carbo Veg, Pulsatilla, Causticum, Sulphur, Hammelis, Lachesis, Calc Carb, Merc Sol.

Uranium Nitricum (Nitrate of Uranium)

Recommended for certain diabetic problems where there is an excess of sugar in the urine (glycosuria).

Urethritis

The condition may be gonorrhoeal in origin or non-specific. Diagnosis and differentiation can usually only be made by microscopy of the discharge which may be thick and creamy-yellow. Cystitis is commonly associated with frequency and burning pains. It is usually sexually-transmitted and can become chronic with scar-tissue formation and an intermittent discharge, or none at all. In gonorrhoeal conditions one course of Penicillin is recommended followed by the homoeopathic remedy to avoid further complications from the infection.

For gonorrhoeal urethritis *Medorrhinum, Merc. Sol, Sulphur.*
For non-specific urethritis, *Petroleum, Silicea, Staphisagria.*

Urinary Difficulties

When little urine is passed the cause may be obstructive as in the infant with phimosis. The outlet is pin-prick in size and the prepuce balloons-out whenever urine is passed. Treatment is surgical and circumcision. Following surgical intervention, the bladder may loose its power of contraction due to irritation from the operation or anaesthetic. For post-operative retention *Causticum 6* is the remedy of choice. Slowness or inability to pass urine may be due to nervousness or impossible when another person is present indicating *Natrum Mur.*

After a stroke there may be paralysis of the bladder nerve supply and *Opium* is recommended. With prostrate problems there is often delay and slowness or a sense of incomplete emptying, requiring *Sabal Serr.*

For the woman the corresponding problem is 'spotting' or slight leaking when rushing, laughing, sneezing or coughing often after damage to the bladder sphincter muscles in childbirth. Remedies include:

Causticum or *Sepia.*

Excessive flow and frequency may be nervous in origin or due to infection, sometimes diabetes. Careful investigation is always necessary.

REMEDIES

Arg. Nit., Ignatia, Sarsparilla.

For stones with 'sticking' pains consider *Berberis.*

Urinary infection is a common recurrent condition (See heading Cystitis). There is the common female problem of frequency, urgency, and burning pains, the water thick or offensive and turbulent.

REMEDIES

Cantharis, Sulphur, Staphisagria, Causticum.

Urtica Urens (Stinging Nettle)

Tincture of the fresh flowering plant. One of the most ancient remedies with a reputation as blood purifier. It is a very useful for scalds and burns, urticaria, rheumatism, insect bites. Recommended by Burnett for gout and as an organ remedy for the Spleen.

The skin is typically red and irritating, itchy, with restlessness marked.

Urticaria

The acute and often recurrent allergic condition, either generalised or more usually local, with several circular patches of raised red wheals on the skin accompanied by itching and frequently malaise. The urticarial eruption may come on very rapidly causing severe anxiety, swelling of the face and throat with malaise. Rarely hospitalisation is required.

Usually it is short lasting, the cause either allergic or from underlying stress and provoked by the most minimal stimulus.

REMEDIES
Astacus (shellfish).
Fragaria (allergy to strawberries).
Pulsatilla (allergy to pork),
Aethusa (allergy to milk).
Also consider *Apis, Arsenicum, Rhus Tox, Urtica, Sulphur.*

Ustilago (Corn Smut, the maize mushroom)

A uterine remedy for congestive menopausal problems and ulceration of the cervix uteri.

Uterine Problems

Careful examination and correction of any misplacement must be carried out at an early stage in treatment. The condition may date from an earlier pregnancy or delivery, sometimes several years previously. Common problems include:
fibroids.

REMEDIES
Fraxinus, Phosphorus, Silicea, Tarentula Hisp.
Flooding or menorrhagia associated from either the menopause or fibroids.

Lachesis, Senecio, Sulphur, Ustilago.
Prolapse of the uterus
Sepia 6.

Uva Ursi (Bearberry)

Recommended for problems of chronic cystisis.

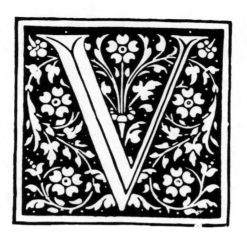

Vaccination

Vaccination is recommended for any virulent infective condition which can totally annihalate the vital reaction of the individual during an epidemic or where there is a special risk. Homoeopathy is required to ensure that the side-effects of vaccination are minimal. For example, Influenza can be of considerable risk to both the elderly and the very young during and epidemic. In such cases when there is a specific vaccine for the specific epidemic it should be used. The homoeopathic alternative is the nosode *Influenzium* which has proved of enormous value in the past when 'flu has reached epidemic proportions. Non-specific vaccination by the 'flu vaccine, unrelated to any specific epidemic is not recommended, the protection minimal, unless there is a specific reason to give it. Similarly plague, typhoid fever, typhus fever, yellow fever should be treated by a conventional specific vaccination programme where there is exposure and wherever the disease is severe or epidemic.

Small pox is not so common now and in most cases vaccination is only recommended routinely for tropical countries where there is a special risk and where it is still endemic. Polio vaccine should be given in its conventional form whenever there is any danger of infection. The whooping cough vaccine does carry a considerable risk to the child and the specific homoeopathic alternative of *Pertussin* is recommended as being effective and without danger of cerebal side-effects.

Homoeopathy is recommended for the side-effects of

269

conventional vaccination. Use *Thuja 6* for local problems of swelling, abscess formation, irritiation of the skin or fever. Give the remedy three times a daily until the condition has cleared and then stop. For conditions of more general nature, where symptoms date since the time of vaccination and never really well since, give *Thuja* in the 30 or 200 potency according to the degree and depth of symptoms.

The final decision on vaccination must be an individual one. There are homoeopathic nosodes available as alternatives for all the common diseases and the final decision as to conventional or homoeopathic nosode must be a personal one, with an intelligent weighing-up of the virulence of the disease at the time and its incidence — either at home or in a country to be visited. When infection or exposure carries a high risk, then use conventional vaccination treating side-effects with homoeopathy in every case unless there are contraindications when homoeopathy can be used as first-line prevention.

Vaginismus

Vaginal spasm during the sexual act. The condition is involuntary and nearly always psychological in origin. Rarely it is associated with pain or inflammation.

REMEDIES
Natrum Mur, Pulsatilla, Platina, Staphisagria, Ignatia.

Valerian Officinalis (Valerian)

The important remedy for excitable psychological states with agitation and restlessness, especially hysterical behaviour and spasms of excitability. Pains are changable and variable, worse for rest and ameliorated by movement (*Rhus Tox.*). There is headache, sore throat, indigestion with nausea, canine hunger, weight loss and diarrhoea. Sighing with tears is frequent. The menstrual pattern is painful and irregular. Restlessness at night with increased agitation and anxiety preventing sleep.

Varicella (Chicken Pox)

The common benign infectious disease of childhood. There is an incubation period of about 13-14 days. Diagnosis is by the typical rash with blisters or vesicles followed by pustules and scab formation but without permanent scarring. The rash typically contains at the same time all three phases of its development. The vesicles are highly infective and in general it is still best to isolate cases from the elderly because of the danger of shingles in that age group. The disease gives a life-long immunity in most cases. Varicella can occasionally occur in the adult when it may pursue a much more severe disagreeable course with malaise, high fever and prostration lasting for several weeks.

REMEDIES

Remedies include the specific varicella nosode both prophylactically and during treatment. *Ant. Tart, Merc Sol, Rhus Tox, Sulphur, Nitric Ac., Psorinum.*

Varicose Veins

The common problem of dilation of and tortuosity of the veins of the lower limb. The leg is swollen, the veins irritating with varicose eczema and ulcer formation in severe or neglected cases. Causes are an increase of back-pressure in the venous system from obstruction or pressure which obstructs the flow and causes damage to the valves and walls of the venous vessels.

The commonest cause is chronic constipation, the heavy, over-loaded large bowel putting all its weight on the long veins of the limbs. Another obvious and frequent cause is pregnancy when the weight of the gravid uterus causes similar obstruction and back-pressure. Obesity aggravates the condition. Other reasons for blockage may be the weight of a fibroid, a cyst or other tumour causing mechanical blockage and weakening of the venous walls.

Piles is another form of varicose problem involving the anal-rectal venous circulation, the causes are basically the same. Bran should be taken regularly in all cases where there is a problem of constipation with a high fibre diet.

REMEDIES

Hammamelis, Pulsatilla, Carbo Veg., Fluoric Acid, Sulphur, Vipera.

Variolinum (Small Pox nosode)

For prevention of the disease when epidemic. Useful in shingles. The skin is infected with acne and pustules, hot and irritated. For the chronic scarring associated with drawn-out cases. Also for chronic acne. (Compare *Thiosinaminum*).

Veratrum Album (White Hellebore)

A major remedy for collapse, lifelessness and shock, but always with extreme chill, pallor and often cyanosis or a mauve-blue tinge to the person. There is profuse sweating, which is drenching but always cold, often icy. Diarrhoea is frequent and watery as with Cholera. Violence, agitation, impulsiveness and restlessness is marked (*Tarentula*). Puerperal psychosis. Suicidal depression Valuable after head injury with concussion (*Helleborus*), headache of a violent pulsating type (*Glonoin*). Severe pre-menstrual tension and irritability.

Veratrum Viride (The White American Hellibore)

Indicated for circulatory problems where there is a general congestion or the danger of an impending cerebral attack or stroke (*Opium*).

Vertigo

The common complaint of dizzyness due to inner-ear disease and disturbance often with nausea and increasing deafness due to degenerative changes of unknown origin. In epilepsy, it may form part of the warning aura of a major attack. With others, in isolation it may reflect a minor petit mal attack or part of temporal-lobe irritation. A common cause is hypertension or raised blood pressure associated with pounding headaches. Often the exact cause is unknown and obscure or psychological and reflects an underlying anxiety or stress problem. Careful diagnosis and investigation is necessary in all cases where response to remedies is slow or unsatisfatory.

REMEDIES
Cocculus, Salicylic Ac., China, Nux Vom, Pulsatilla, Natrum Mur, Sulphur, Conium, Spigelia.

Viburnum Op (High Cranberry)

The menstrual remedy for dysmenorrhoa where the flow is of brief duration. Cramping pains are characteristic — of stomach, intestine and uterus. Miscarriage of the third month, bleeding, pain at ovulation, are the other indications.

Viburnum Tinus (Lauristus)

The cardiac or respiratory remedy with oppression in the chest and shortness of breath. The patient holds a hand to the heart in a gesture of weakness and anxiety. The pupils may be irregular.

Vinca Minor (Periwinkle)

The valuable scalp remedy for lifeless hair, hair loss, patchy alopoecia, and itchy scalp eczema. Itching,eczema, infected areas generally with hypersensitivity of the part affected and redness.

Viola Tricolour (Pansy)

Recommended for chronic skin condition with infected eczemas or impetigo. There is a pusy discharge and severe irritation, Enuresis.

Vipera Redi (Viper Venom)

The remedy for severe phlebitis with venous engorgement, irritation. Phlebitis, varicose ulcers.

Viscum Alb. (Mistletoe)

For lack of vital reaction or collapse, The pulse is slow — blood pressure lowered, with oppression and shortness of breath on the least movement or exertion. Exhaustion. A remedy for the most desperate and extreme conditions.(Compare *Veratrum Alb* — the remedy lacks the chill and extreme sweating of *Veratrum*).

Visual Fatigue

Eye strain due to excessive reading or close work, often in poor light conditions and always better for rest. There may be a need for new spectacles or the ocular lens is unable to focus correctly from disease or due to age. Cataract with misty vision may be another factor. Psychological features can also play a role in some instances.

REMEDIES

Euphrasia, Ruta, Gelsemium, Alumina, Calc. Carb. Zinc. Met.

Vital Energy

The inherited vital principle or life force, present throughout life but undermined by disease, miasm or stress. It is the first part of the person affected when disease occurs and causes the very early symptoms of malaise, fatigue and irritability or lack of interest which precede the development of symptoms — often by several months. Vital force attaches itself in a protective way to the disease process in order to bind and contain it protecting the vital organs. The homoeopathic remedies in the higher potencies act first and foremost upon vital energy, supporting its protective functioning role. Vital energy is usually the first area to be relieved by homoeopathy as the remedies act at the centre initially and the malaise, jaded indifference, fatigue and lack of energy is relieved long before more specific symptoms, according to the law of cure.

Vomiting

Always a serious symptom which may or may not be accompanied by nausea. Every case needs careful consideration and investigation of underlying causative factors. A surgical condition must always be excluded. Causes vary considerably, with emotional factors common in the child and certain adolescents (anorexia). In hysterical illness it may be a worrying symptom at any age often defying all treatment and diagnosis . Other common causes are dietary indiscretions when the cause is usually obvious, the effects short lasting. Alcoholism is a familiar cause. Other causes include peptic ulcer, hiatus hernia, acute infective conditions of childhood and the central nervous system as meningitis. Blood may be vomited — several pints of fresh blood or mixed with food and only partially digested. These conditions require urgent surgery as too vomiting from intestinal obstruction whatever the cause. The problem should be under medical care and if there is doubt, investigations carried out carefully to clarify underlying reasons for the symptom.
REMEDIES
Nux. Vom, Pulsatilla, Natrum Mur, Phosphorus, Aethusa, Cocculus, Ipecac, Arsenicum.

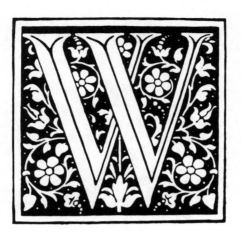

Warts

The common viral skin infection, occuring on any part of the body with outgrowths of a rough irregular type which may bleed or spread by contact to adjacent skin areas. In general they should not be interferred with and usually there is a good response to homoeopathy. Large warts on the sole of the feet need special attention if enlarging or bleeding and may require surgery. Anal or genital warts with a stem or cauliflower surface often indicate a sycotic miasmic condition and require special consideration and thorough treatment by the homoeopathic method.

REMEDIES
Causticum, Dulcamara, Ant. Crud, Thuja, Nitric Acid, Fluoric Acid.

Weir, Sir John, G.C.V.O., M.D. (1879-1971)

The eminent physician and homoeopath to the royal family and late queen of Norway. Weir qualified in Glasgow in 1906 and was immediately influenced by Gibson-Miller, who treated a condition of boils, which had not responded to conventional treatments, with such success, that he became his homoeopathic mentor. With the support of Tyler in 1908 he studied with both Allen and Kent at the Chicago Hering Homoeopathic College, returning to become physician to the London Homoeopathic Hospital in 1910 and Compton-Burnett Professor of Materia Medica in 1911. He was an impressive advocate of the single dose and of non-interference with any aggravation-response by the patient. President of the faculty in 1923, his lectures, addresses and articles are numerous with a directness and simplicity which is refreshing. In spite of his eminence, Weir was always regarded as a man of enormous humility.

Wesselhoef, Conrad, M.D. (1834-1904)

The American homoeopath, active in the last half of the 19th C. His major writing contributions include.
1872 *The cause of contention between the old and the new*
1880 *The method of our work*
1881 *A plea for a standard of the attenuated dosage*
1883 *Is the homoeopathy of Hahnemann the homoeopathy of today?*
1883 *The law of the similars*
1887 *How to study the materia medica*
Also translator of Hahnemann's *Organon in 1876.*

Wheeler, Charles Edwin, M.D. (1868-1946)

The Australian homoeopath, trained at Barts and staff member of the London Homoeopathic Hospital from 1904. President of the British Homoeopathic Society and of the International League, he was a stimulating writer and lecturer.
His major writings include:
Introduction to the Principles and Practise of Homoeopathy
Fools or Knaves – a defence of homoeopathy
Chronic Diseases, written with E. Bach
He was also involved in a major translation of the *Organon.*

Woods, Harold Fergie-, M.D. (1883-1961)

The homoeopath who was a student of Kent in Chicago with Weir on a Tyler scholarship in 1908. He returned to support the case for high potency prescribing and the single dosage. Physician at the early Children's Homoeopathic Dispensary in Shepherd's Bush, founded by Roberson Day in 1920 and later amalagamated with the London Homoeopathic Hospital in 1935. Consultant to the London Hospital, he was a founder member of the International League in 1925. In spite of increasing blindness he was active for homoeopathy throughout and a gifted prescriber and physician.

Whooping Cough

A highly infectious condition of infancy and childhood marked by attacks of paroxysmal coughing leading to blueness of the face as the larynx and respiratory muscles go into spasm followed by a long, deep breath causing the characteristic whoop — which is diagnostic. Paroxysms of coughing lead to vomiting or congestion with nose bleeds. The condition may last weeks and often follows a drawn-out course. It is mainly of danger to the very youngest child and in recent years the illness has largely followed a milder pattern.

REMEDIES

Pertussin prophylactically from six months, unless there is contact when it can be given earlier. The nosode should be repeated every six months until the age of five. During acute illness give *Pertussin,* and consider *Drosera, Ipecac, Ant Tart, Belladonna, Carbo Veg, Arnica, Nux Vom, Phosphorous.*

Worms

These occur as either Round Worms (Ascarides), Threadworms (Oxyures), Tapeworms (Taenia). Of these, by far the commonest is the threadworm. See separate headings.

Wounds

In all cases stop the bleeding by local pressure or a tourniquet applied intermittantly. Shock must be treated by keeping the patient warm and giving *Arnica* or *Veratrum Alb.* If more severe. Repeat *Arnica* every few minutes until there is a response. Careful cleaning of the area is essential when hospitalisation is not considered necessary or in unavailable. All foreign matter must be removed, the wound cleaned with *Calendula* and when large, or in a cosmetic area, suturing should be carried out. A clean sterile dressing must be applied over the *Calendula.* Tetanus vaccination is required for a dirty wound. When in doubt the patient should be taken to the nearest hospital casualty department, homoeopathy acting as an additional supportive therapy to conventional treatments.

REMEDIES

Arnica (shock),

Aconitum (restlessness and agitation),
China (for loss of blood),
Veratrum Alb. (collapse),
Ledum (punctured wounds),
Hypericum (nerve damage and shooting pains),
Arsenicum (for infection).

Wyethia Helenoides (Poison Weed)

Recommended for severe cases of chronic dry cough, hay fever, pharyngitis.

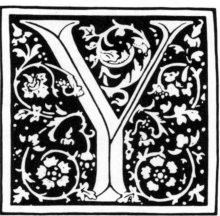

XYZ

X-Ray (ethanol exposed to x-ray)

For any conditions, particularly of the skin, but also of any organ of the body which has never functioned since exposure to x-ray diagnosis or treatment.

Zincum Metallum (Zinc)

One of Hahnemann's anti-psora remedies for chronic conditions of agitiation and restlessness with nervous twitching or convulsions. The condition typically involves the lower limbs and feet with 'fidgety feet', and oversensitivity to the least noise of stimulus.

It includes paralysis and meningitis.

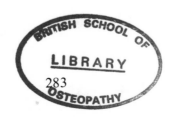

BRITISH SCHOOL OF LIBRARY 283 OSTEOPATHY

By the same Author
Homoeopathic Medicine
The Homoeopathic Treatment of Emotional Illness
Understanding Homoeopathy

The British School of Osteopathy

* 4 1 5 0 *

This book is to be returned on or before
the last date stamped below.

- 8 JAN. 1996

7 FEB.

MAY 1998

An
Encyclopaedia
of Homoeopathy

A complete survey of the homoeopathic method and
approach in alphabetical form including the history,
philosophy, major personalities, remedies and illnesses,
written by a doctor with 25 years experience of holistic
medicine.

SMITH, TREVOR

An encyclopaedia of
Homoeopathy